MW00812110

THE KAMA SUTRA

THE PRACTICAL GUIDE TO MIND-BLOWING
ORGASMS WITH THE KAMA SUTRA, TANTRIC SEX
TEACHINGS, AND CLIMAX ENHANCING SEX
POSITIONS

KELLY ANDERSON

CONTENTS

© Copyright 2019 - All rights reserved.

It is not legal to reproduce, duplicate, or transmit any part of this document in either electronic means or in printed format. Recording of this publication is strictly prohibited and any storage of this document is not allowed unless with written permission from the publisher except for the use of brief quotations in a book review.

INTRODUCTION

Before there was language, society or even consciousness, there was sex. It is the fundamental building block to life—reproduction, continuation, and existence. Sex is within humans as an animalistic, biological imperative. But then, one day, and for reasons unknown to science or religion, humanity switched on. In a moment, biological imperative had a companion: desire.

Over thousands and thousands of years, humanity perfected this desire through each generation—developing, improving, and communicating to the next. But in many Western cultures, that stopped. Sex became sin, something to be ashamed of and hide. Any expression of lust and desire was dissuaded through punishment and social forces.

Generations passed on minimal, if any, information to the next.

Contrarily, in the East, sex was not seen as a selfish or masochistic act. It was simply a part of life in the vein of business, love, food. It was both pleasure and power, practiced and lived within the context of the larger society. It had its problems, but it was built on a level of consciousness rather than morality. One man, Vātsyāyana, recognized its value and decided to do something good about it. He wrote three books. The subject of this book, the *Kama Sutra*, speaks to the world of love and sex.

But he did not do it alone. More than anything, the *Kama Sutra* is the combined knowledge of hundreds of generations and thousands of years of human experience. It is a point in time before sex transitioned in the West from pleasure to sin. More than sex, the *Kama Sutra* depicts love and life as it was then and will be for all of humanity. About twenty percent of the book is about sex—but that twenty percent represents thousands of years of knowledge, experimentation, and perfection for multiple cultures and their people. The best part?

It has been translated into English. After generations of disinformation and shame, people in the West can access the information built over thousands of years. Westerners can reset through education and under-standing, revolutionize their personal sex life overnight simply through shifting a mindset and understanding the ideas behind the *Kama Sutra*.

This book condenses that knowledge into a few, concise chapters. The specifics of positions and an understanding of how to perform them will make your sex life better, of course. It is like being a magi-cian who learns more card tricks. The act will get better once you can spice it up with some new tricks. But if you want to enchant someone, if you want to change their perspective on love and life in one night with amazing, self-expressive sex, there is more to learn than a few moves.

But those moves are worth going into. This book will review a variety of positions and situations, from the intimacies associated with good foreplay to the tried and tested positions for sex between a man and a woman. Not only have these positions been ranked and organized based on difficulty, they encompass information passed down through the *Kama Sutra* in conjunction with modern approaches to sex.

These ideals of love and sex extend into the Tantric

realm. Tantric practices, much like the *Kama Sutra* in general, have been reduced down to ideas of sex and the maximization of sexual pleasure. While the sexual aspects of Tantric are discussed, the role of Tantric practices in a relationship is explored more deeply. The goal of Tantric relationships is to have a unified consciousness—something achieved through deep meditation and connection to each other in an intimate setting.

This book will give you the tools you need to become a better, more generous, come complete lover. Beyond lessons on how to give love and pleasure, there are also those about how to receive love. How to let go in the moment, falling back into the ecstasy that is pleasure of all kinds. This extends outside the bedroom as well, into the relationships you hold as complete units rather than only the delicacies of the bedroom. As important as sex and physical and spiritual connection are to a relationship, they are only a part. Some of these teachings will help you to inject your relationship with an adrenaline shot. Others will advise, in that specific moment, you do the complete opposite. It is up to you to have the wisdom to know when and where is appropriate to apply each of these tools. Because, at the end of the day, they are tools.

Women do not have a magic button to press that gives them an orgasm involuntarily. Men are not lustful beasts. There is nuance, there is love, and there is a need to navigate these. This book, before anything else, will help you to understand a different way to approach love, lust, sex, manipulation, and deception. Not only that, it will expand your mind into the potential for a deeper, awesome connection with your partner that can be witnessed and experienced regularly.

Sex is more than that moment. It's everything around it as well. From foreplay to the mentality, positions, and toys, sex can be all-encompassing. It is immensely powerful, and you have that power. This book will help you unlock its fullest potential. Beyond that single aspect of a relationship, it will also grant a glimpse into a different approach to relationships and love. Enter with a curious and open mind; there are many things to learn!

MINDSET OF THE KAMA SUTRA

*B*efore any diagrams or descriptions of specific foreplay techniques, there is an all too critical sexual mindset that needs to be addressed. More than a book articulating sexual satisfaction, the Kama Sutra is a piece of philosophy —the positions, methods, and systems in it will not work without an understanding of that philosophy. For that, we need to look back briefly and outline some of the cultural pieces that are holding you back from having good sex.

Vātsyāyana, a philosopher of ancient India, is cred-ited as the author of the *Kama Sutra*, but the ideas were not new. He had collected hundreds of years of spiritual wisdom. Around the same time as he was on the bank of the River Ganges writing about how to have oral sex, the Equinimical Council in Rome had made a decree against sex. They banned oral and anal sex outright, saying it was immoral, wrong, and punishable by death. In that world, the Catholic church deemed pleasure as a sin, something wrong, something to be treated with malice. That was the birth of modern sexual morality—the idea that there were right and wrong forms of sex. If sex was not in the context of marriage in the name of having a child, it was wrong. How much of that sentiment has remained in our society today?

Compare that with the origins of the *Kama Sutra*. The *Kama Sutra* is one of three books working to describe life. It is less a book about sex and more a piece working to describe acts of love, passion, desire, and spirituality. It was written in a period with a completely different foundation for reality. A key piece of adopting their teachings is under-standing and absorbing the base upon which they are built. These teachings go beyond the bedroom, emphasizing the importance of sexual energy as energy of creation. The *Kama Sutra* speaks of sexual energy as a force of nature, primal and deliberate, something to be expressed and understood in multiple arenas. Moments of passion or arousal, inspiration or creativity, excitement or interest, all come from the same place. To limit the teachings of the *Kama Sutra* to sexual exploration is limiting the entire collective wisdom of civilizations long forgotten.

But, we're going to do it anyway. The modern view of sex in western societies is very limited for a few reasons. There are two things specifically that need to be addressed.

1. SEX IS NOT THE CUSTOMS LINE AT THE AIRPORT.

You've just gotten off the plane, tired, hungry, and excited to visit a new country. After waiting in line for a while, you walk up to the immigration officer. They ask you a few questions, maybe take your picture. Then, they stamp your passport. Once the ink transfers from the dated stamp to the passport, you are definitively in the country. You don't need to ask the immigration officer if you're in, nor do you have to give anyone anything else. You're fine, you're in, it is binary. Like flipping a coin, either you're in or you're out.

In the *Kama Sutra*, sex is not a binary of good or bad, right or wrong, orgasm or no-gasm. Rather, sex is like color. There is red hot sex: fiery, passionate, fast, intense sex. But imagine a world where you only saw the color red. Would you not miss the blue and white of the ocean? Or the browns and greens smattered throughout a forest? Sure, the red hot is good. But is it good constantly? It loses its touch after a while. Things need to shift. But when people look at sex as a positive or a negative, they define good and bad sex binarily. They draw a line in the sand somewhere and say, "This is good, this is bad, and I need to be on the good side". The consequence of doing that is you lose that ability to taste the different colors, and you're left with the pressure to accomplish forms for all parties involved rather than an ability to enjoy it.

Sex is not right or wrong, good or bad. It is pleasure distilled down to human experience. Focus on the pleasure, desire, and energy rather than an arbitrary idea of success or failure.

2. THERE IS NO CAMERA.

Piecing together where modern sexual expectations come from is not difficult. We need only consider two factors: porn and Hollywood. And while those are great for getting people into the movie theaters or a long list of Trojan horse viruses, they are not great examples for sex. In fact they aren't even great for the people involved.

"Well, it is a little bit," you might say. Nope, not even a little bit. Think of the hottest, steamiest sex scene from any movie. It wasn't exactly intimate. It can't have been. Not only are you observing as a consumer of the final production, but think of the number of people involved in its making. In fact filming one sex scene usually involved between 7 and 13 people off set. Often times, significant others are also observing. A 15-second sex scene with different shots might take more than six hours to shoot, typically with a lunch break in between. Male actors are often wearing "modesty socks" the entire time, if they aren't both wearing jeans. But that's Hollywood. Porn is real!

Porn is actually more misleading than Hollywood shoots. Ten minutes of porn, on average, take 4 hours to shoot. The job of a porn star is not to enjoy the body of another person, it's to look right at the camera. Often the positions that look right on camera are not comfortable or attempts at pleasure in the slightest. The job of the performers is to still look like they're having the best sex of their entire lives after four, five, or six hours of shooting. They're fatigued, tired, and often having sex with people they would rather not.

For most of the western world, the things that have informed how to have sex are completely fabricated performances designed to look good rather than feel good. Sex is not a look good or bad situation, it's a pleasure bar. Before you read anything else about the *Kama Sutra*, it is of unparalleled importance that this is understood: *the things in porn, the things in Hollywood blockbusters,* **are designed to look good rather than feel good.** The goal of sex is pleasure, not to be photographed while you do it.

The *Kama Sutra* is not merely a list of positions to add to your personal repertoire, ready to whip out at a moment's notice. Doing these positions and applying these philosophies with the porn/Hollywood mentality **will completely undermine the positions.**

You are not a performer. You're a person. From a physical perspective, there are things you like, curiosities, and fantasies swirling around in your head. At a spiritual level, there are connections to build and evolve with a consenting partner who is as interested in doing the same with you.

The Kama Sutra Mindset

The 'Birds and the Bees' story is one way of thinking about and introducing sex to children, and it holds up for reproduction. If you are only having sex to have a child, great. But the expectation for sex has outgrown the restrictions of 300 AD Catholic Equinimical Council. Sex is supposed to be pleasurable in every way—physical, mental and spiritual all in one act. It builds a bridge between two people, beyond the logical and rational, like a fast lane to the soul of another person. Of course, there are things we can all do better to make sex feel more pleasurable, but they can only be achieved through a different mindset than is common in Western erotica. How does the sex in the *Kama Sutra* differ in mindset?

1. CONFIDENCE IS KEY

Sure, for a job interview, personal confidence is very important. But the *Kama Sutra* takes this idea to a completely new level. Confidence in yourself is of minimal importance. Sexual prowess and experience mean nothing in this arena. Throw them out the window. **The first job of a sexual partner is to make the other feel confident.** This means helping them overcome fears and insecurities leading up to, during, and after the act. The other person's confidence is the most important part of a sexual interaction.

2. PERSISTENCE AND EFFORT

Better sex does not come easy. It is one of life's pleasures that is worth working on. Sex is a dance that begins before ever getting to the bedroom. The *Kama Sutra* suggests manipulation and deception are as legitimate functions of sex as honesty and forwardness.

It argues further against the ideals of classical Romanticism in a few ways, suggesting there is no "one" person for any of us. Beyond the idea of the one, there is an ocean of people looking to develop and grow. The necessity of the individual is to take the burden of responsibility upon themselves rather than weigh it upon the fate of the universe. All too often, the ideals of destiny and fate allow people to wrongly absolve themselves of responsibility. These things take work! Reading this book is the first step to that study, but it is not the last. Invest time into the things you want and you shall reap the rewards.

Sow seeds only once then neglect them, and there will be no benefit.

The *Kama Sutra* asks that the individual, specifically, a man, evolve with the reality they find themselves in. Never stop, simply shift and recalibrate, figuring out what works along the way. If men and women were left to their own devices, they would not come together. Adaptive effort, attention, and persistence will overcome most obstacles to love.

3. CONNECTION OVER CONSUMPTION

Many similarities between the love described in the *Kama Sutra* can be seen in Socrates' *Symposium* and even Chrisitan doctrine within the Bible. An expanding mindset within the *Kama Sutra* is that there are four different types of love: love by habit, love by imagination, mutual love, and unnamed love.

Love by habit is the easiest and most available of the loves. It is love through action, constant and continuous action. From there, there is love through the imagination, which is fabricated upon ideas and wishes rather than realized physical reality. Mutual love is a shared recognition of the other as an individual who loves you. These are powerful forms of love, yet the *Kama Sutra* strongly implies that unnamed love, a love obvious to all outside observers yet hidden from the lovers, is the most powerful of all loves. Why is that?

When the two lovers do not see it, they stumble upon it with no expectations. Expectation kills relationships, love, and sex appeal. In the absence of its burden, lovers can flourish and express themselves honestly. They can be confident within themselves, find meaning in a newfound pleasure, and overcome obstacles to build something authentic. Two individuals can connect with more force because nothing is detracting from that sensation.

There is no good or bad form of love—as the *Kama Sutra* expresses it. However, the larger lesson is to abandon expectations. When you enter the bedroom, do it wide-eyed and ready to experience rather than entering with a to-do list. It is a more pleasurable experience and empowers the juxtaposition of light, yet deep love to unravel.

At the end of the day, the *Kama Sutra* is a book about a small piece of life feeding into and contributing to the whole. This is a product of its time. To use it as a way to legitimize the modern, porno-driven method to having sex is to miss the entire point. Sex to these people was not a taboo subject, nor was it held with the same esteem and focus our culture has for it. It was simply something else—another part of life. That is not to say the benefits of the *Kama Sutra* cannot be applied to the world around us and within the context of the 21st century. But to do so requires a shift in mindset. There is consistency between men and women; the author of the *Kama Sutra* and the people he lived among were no different physically. But they had a separate mindset, a different set of guiding principles that they applied to sex.

It was not the only set of principles. Every culture has its own form of erotica and pleasure. But it is different. In the same way that going to different restaurants is a pleasurable experience, having sex should always include fresh and more pleasurable experiences. The ten books of the *Kama Sutra* dives into many specifics about finding women or men, methods for manipulation and interactions, and aphrodisiacs. Included within the bounds are guides to interacting within the society of the time, finding the best ways to develop sexual relationships into marriages, and many ideas that would infuriate any feminist. It was a different time in a different society. But the collective wisdom of multiple, ancient societies and their experiences with the timeless themes of love and sex is valuable in spite of those differences.

The extraction of sexual wisdom from this base philosophy is possible on the condition that you align with the mindset of the time. Adopting anti-feminist rhetoric or the morality of culture hundreds of years old is not required. However, internalizing a resistance to judgment and classification, a desire for pleasure over congratulations, and a longing for connection within another person beyond the intellectual: those are ideas worth absorbing into life beyond the bedroom as well. For now, though, let us explore the intricacies and techniques behind foreplay.

In the next chapter, we're going to apply the philosophies and ideas behind the *Kama Sutra*'s sexual experience to modern foreplay in Western cultures.

2

ESSENTIAL FOREPLAY TECHNIQUES

*I*magine you're sitting at a bar. A couple walks up beside you—a man and a woman. Neither of them has any problems with drinking, they simply want to relax on a first date. So, naturally, they both casually order a drink to sip and enjoy.

The man gets a smooth beer. It is so easy to drink that he ends up ordering another, and another, and another until he gets to where he wants to be. The woman orders a tall glass of straight vodka. She has been slowly sipping as the man sprints through beers, but nothing seems to affect her. The man can drink beers all night, but it takes time, patience and willpower to get through an entire glass of straight vodka.

This is roughly how male and female orgasms occur relative to one another. For men, it is relatively quick to get excited and to orgasm—but, for women, it takes time and effort, like a balancing act of psychological, physiological and social pressures in one moment. For all the differences between the two, there is one base commonality—the importance of foreplay.

Imagine that same first date, but after two drinks the man hopped down on one knee, professed his love for the woman, and asked her to marry him. What would the woman's reaction be? In a modern dating situation where years may pass before even considering the question, how uncomfortable and rushed would that feel? The same notion applies to sex. Foreplay is the build up to the climax, the runway to the plane. If it is too short, there was never a chance to take off.

Foreplay makes sex better for both parties involved. In multiple studies, scientists found that foreplay builds up a more enjoyable and pleasurable orgasm, helps men last longer while having sex, and can even make the male erection larger (in the case of oral stimulation vs. self stimulation). For a woman, foreplay is a requirement for pleasure. It works to get the three different parts of sex, physiological, psychological and social, on the same page and working to the same goal: climax. If all three are not present, it is very difficult for a woman to climax. Foreplay erodes the barriers to pleasure over, ideally, 18 minutes.

Lovemaking vs. Sex

Desire is a natural expression of the self that applies to things and dreams as much as it does to sex and pleasure. Sex is great at providing pleasure, both physical and mental. However, there is a line in the sand where the sex becomes something different. When sex becomes vulnerable with the expressed hope for connection to the partner, a deep and intimate walk in emotional tandem down to the core of each other's being, sex can transition to lovemaking, should you let it.

lovemaking is characterized by that intimacy. Where sex is focused on pleasure, climax, and fun, lovemaking is a deep openness that spawns within those moments. The focus shifts from the climax to the foreplay, but it moves beyond the sensations of touch. It incorporates taste and smell. Rather than dirty talk, there are gentle whispers of affirmation and love that come through. There are conversations about how much each person cares about the other with eyes locked. Intense vulnerability and emotional openness grant access to a spiritual experience and nourishment of the soul beyond the physical pleasures of the self. There is authenticity through honesty to it that is difficult to achieve through sex alone. And, at the end of it all, you may decide an orgasm is not even worth it. That is not the point. It is an exercise in spiritual openness.

It is still, at a physical level, occurring within the body, which means that, as someone making love or having sex, certain access points allow for the experience of greater pleasure. These are called erogenous zones.

The Seven Erogenous Zones

There are seven specific spots of the body that might be a little more receptive. Not only are these described in great detail in the Kama Sutra, but their existence has also backed up by and explored thoroughly by modern science. Accessing each of these is a matter of touch. Kisses, nibbles, pecks, and licks all work to stimulate these hotbeds of sexual energy. For men, in order from greatest to least pleasurable, they are:

1. Penis
2. Mouth and Lips
3. Scrotum
4. Neck + Nape of Neck
5. Nipples
6. Perineum/Taint
7. Feet

For women, there exists a similar seven:

1. clitoris
2. Vagina
3. Cervix
4. Mouth and Lips
5. Neck + Nape of Neck
6. Breasts + Nipples
7. Ears

There are a few disputed points as well—many men may not derive pleasure from the nipples while others enjoy the feet. For women, it is common to hear the inside of the wrist as a disputed eighth and ninth zone. Regardless, these generalizations are to be explored within the context of foreplay. Reading the body language and reaction of your partner, as well as communicating, is critical to add to the pleasure road map of erogenous zones. What better way to explore these zones than with a kiss?

Kissing

The first kiss is the start of every great romance; kissing holds the utmost importance within a relationship, yet often it is limited to pecks. Outside of the *Kama Sutra*, Vātsyāyana ended up describing in detail over 5,000 different types of kisses. How many have you tired? There are virtually infinite iterations of kisses that can be tried and experimented. In fact a whole field of study called philematology has been dedicated to the craft in what must be an HR nightmare within any university. The *Kama Sutra* also explicitly states where to deliver the kisses: the forehead, the eyes, the cheeks, the throat, the bosom, the breasts, the lips, and the interior of the mouth. Each has its own set of kisses with variables of pressure, tongue involvement, lip pursing, and breath. For example, a kiss on the eyelids should be gentle and firm, while a kiss on the lips or mouth might enjoy some variable tongue action or licking.

Nevertheless, here are a few interesting permutations from the *Kama Sutra*:

1. *The Contact Kiss*: Lightly touch the tongue to the other person's lips, outlining the part of the mouth, before kissing it gently.

2. *The Bent Kiss*: Toss your head back and let your partner kiss on and under the chin, into the neck or Adam's apple, and eventually make their way one direction or the other.

3. *The Curling Kiss*: When kissing a woman's breast, trail the tongue gently under the breast, trailing to the nipple.

4. *The Delicate Kiss*: From the nape of the neck, gently purse your lips and nibble without the teeth, like planting small seeds into their back. Combine this with the warmth of your breath.

5. *The Metaphor Kiss*: kissing an object or body part in the presence of the lover, insinuating the kiss was meant for them. This is described in the *Kama Sutra* through the use of a child, which is obviously inappropriate today. Objects work better in the 21st century.

With all things, kissing is something that is best personalized. How does your partner react to biting of the wrist or licking of the ear? Foreplay is a chance to figure out the little ticks of a person if it is the first time together. If you enter foreplay with knowledge of the person from past experiences, changing up the kiss can be a great way to explore further and keep them guessing. After all, there are over 5,000 written down. Even with such a grand number, there are still intricacies that you can personally explore with your partner. Experiment, keep them on their toes, and know that options exist for new forms of kissing. Although it is one of the most effective and fun foreplay forms, kissing is not the only in existence.

Foreplaying

At its core, foreplay is finding pleasurable, creative ways to communicate a single idea: "I want you". Good foreplay considers context, personality, and rhythm during the act. But it should never begin in the bedroom. Remember, sex is a psychological game as well. It means starting hours before and miles away from the bed.

Before the Bedroom (Or Other Area)

A romance novel is often 300 pages of will they, won't they leading up to one final moment. Romance is probing that question—building tension and suspense through anticipation. There are many, many ways to do this, so get creative! Today, this takes many forms. Believe it or not, "sexts", the act of injecting sexual innuendo or fantasy into text messages, is the easiest way to go about this. Simply being away from one another with the anticipation, fantasizing about what will happen when you reconnect, can be enough. It is directing their attention to you and the amazing, mind-blowing pleasure they will experience later. But there are many creative ways to do it, so have fun with it! The key is that something needs to be restricting your ability to do something about the desire. Seducing your partner, new and vibrant or experienced and practiced, is about playing the game of anticipation and tension. Build up, and release. Here are a few ideas to get you started:

1. Calendar updates
2. Act like you don't know one another
3. Take charge

There are a few things to consider. Where you are can affect the mood and type of sex outright. Sex in a broom closet during a bridesmaid speech is very different from having a bedroom for the entire night. The mood flows through the physical space as much as it does through the actions of each person. So, when possible, manipulate the space. This means addressing things like light, sound, smell, temperature, and time beforehand. Everything should be in service to the pleasure. The light should never be too overwhelming, the music, not distracting or out of touch, the smell soothing and the temperature consistent. The manipulation of time works in favor of the excitement, be it a guarantee or a lack thereof.

Early touch is electric. But remember that in foreplay, it is all in service to the buildup of tension. This can be a nurturing touch, such as a shave or wash, which can work wonders on deepening an existing connection. More traditional flirting like footsie under the table, stealing a kiss or sneaking hands can do wonders for the desire of the other. But more than anything, it must be in service to a larger tension, probing and prodding rather than fulfilling.

In the Act

It's on. As we spoke about before, do not skip the foreplay and jump right into the sex. Pressure equals pleasure. Let the pressure mount as long as you can, then act for a more pleasurable and satisfying experience. There are many, many ways this can happen, involve chocolates and food, a striptease, or a massage are all great ways as well. In conjunction with those, oral sex is one of the best ways to get a partner going. But in this section, let's focus on the specific acts you may not be paying enough attention to that drive both men and women wild.

For Women

It is said a man's word is his bond. This is not limited to business or politics. In fact it extends to the bedroom as well. Say what you're going to do then do it. This is a very, very easy way to drive her wild and increase that tension even further. However, whereas some women like when you take control, others don't want to hear your voice at all. There is no one rule. Regardless, communication not only makes for better sex, it works to stimulate that psychological side of the experience. Keep in mind that the bulk of communication is non-verbal.

The delicate, careful licking and kissing of a woman's breast are extremely sensual. It touches on hundreds of thousands of nerve endings both in and around the nipple. Do not neglect the breast in the name of the nipple. Find your way around, invitingly kissing and probing throughout the area to find her spots.

Kissing and licking the body, in general, extends beyond the breast. Kissing is the easy, low-cost method for getting a woman to beg for you. It should extend through the seven erogenous zones and into the nooks and crannies of the body, arms and underarms, inner thighs, and pelvis. In combination with these, the breath and saliva work in tandem to shift the temperatures of different areas.

For Men

Before kisses fly, women have a special ability to flip the roles and take charge. Small acts like pushing them on the bed before taking their clothes off, leading him to the bedroom, or a small tease can work wonders. Anything that gives the sense that you're in control of the situation can be very stimulating for the man. Sometimes the opposite, being submissive, can work to positive effect. Asking for him to come into the bedroom, telling him you need him, and other forms of begging often make him more than willing to oblige.

Many of the same rules for women apply to men. Licking and kissing gently around the body to find points of congested tension does wonders, especially around the pelvis or neck. These are places that men store a lot of energy and pressure. A kiss or nibble in these spaces can drive them wild.

Biting

Biting, grabbing and scratching are all great ways to express a craving for your partner. It separates the inexperienced from those who have studied up. This is known as odaxelagnia and is either a hit or a miss. The key is a mixture of pressure and timing, but it is one of the easiest and most accepted forms of sexual sadism. It is best to focus on the erogenous zones for biting, while the back, buttocks, and legs are all great places to scratch. The *Kama Sutra* specifically outlines a few different types of biting:

1. *The Hidden Bite*: soft, only shown by the slight redness of the skin, often scattered or on the lips
2. *The Swollen Bite*: presses the skin down on both sides, typically around the ear
3. *The Point*: a light, little bite on a specific part of the skin, using two teeth
4. *The Line of Points*: form a circle of points around, near or on an erogenous zone. These are best applied to the throat, armpit, and joints.

5. *The Coral and the Jewels*: biting with your full mouth to create an ornamental indentation with your teeth. These also are best dispersed around the throat, armpit, and joints.

6. *The Broken Cloud*: small bites that form light, cloud looking marks. On a woman, this is usually done around the breast and nipples.

7. *The Biting of the Boar*: the biting of the boar is a harder, intense bite in a moment of intensity. Be careful to regulate to your partner's pain threshold, but it can be extremely intimate. Typically, this is reserved for the shoulders or breasts.

Biting is a great way to shock the system in a moment of passion, forcing the body to react to a quick burst of unexpected pain only to crash down into a wave of pleasure. There is one more way to build the tension of foreplay—something that runs completely counter to biting and scratching.

Massaging and Oils

A prerequisite for pleasure is relaxation. The juxta-position between relaxation and sexual tension is best embodied through a sensual massage. These are not Thai massages complete with wrestling moves or intense pounding on your partner's back. These are gentle, soft massages designed to elicit stimulation and squirming more than breaking down a knot.

The key to an erotic massage is the use of oil. Which type is highly dependent on the person receiving the massage, so ask and experiment. It is important to take care when applying oil, making sure it is safe to do so for all parties. This is especially important if the oil has been slightly heated before application. Studies show that certain aphrodisiac properties of different oils affect men and women differently; keeping that distinction in mind is important when choosing the proper oil. For women: clary sage, lavender, sandalwood, and ylang-ylang are preferred aphrodisiac oils. For men, *Carpolobia*, *Eurycoma longifolia*, and *Casimiroa edulis* oils provide greater sexual stimulation. However, the distinction between these oils is minimal compared to the massage practice you're using in conjunction with them.

There are many forms of massages, but there are seven main forms that are great for men and women.

1. DUO OR FOUR HANDS MASSAGE

This massage involves two people laboring over the receiver's body, meticulously massaging every part of the body. It involves oil on the masseuses and the receiver, typically very time consuming and meticulous. It is often an overwhelming visual and physical experience for the receiver enjoyed over a long period.

2. NURU MASSAGE

Nuru, meaning "slippery" in Japanese, is also known as the body-to-body massage. This involves a masseuse taking all of their clothes off, applying an odorless, tasteless oil to both them and the giver, then rubbing their body on the receiver. The goal of a *Nuru* massage is to get the widest possible contact, often leading directly into intercourse. The key to a *Nuru* massage is the oil, a specialty oil made from seaweed, which is typically premade.

3. YONI OR VAGINAL MASSAGE

A *Yoni* massage is a full body Tantric massage that culminates in the massage of the vagina, the G-spot, and the clitoris. It is often used as an exercise to help women go through a transformative spiritual experience. It is important to create a relaxing space that allows her to enter a completely calm state, focusing on the vagina in conjunction with the entire body.

4. LINGAM OR PENIS MASSAGE

This massage specifically focuses on the natural simulations within the penis, including the shaft, testicles, perineum/taint, and external prostate. Similar to the *yoni* massage, it involves a full body rub and massage that then culminates in a massage of the penis.

5. PROSTATE MASSAGE

For men, the prostate is known as an emotional, sexual, and sacred part of the body. Not only is it connected to physical sensations, but there are also many psychological pressures that contribute to pressure buildup in the area. A massage stimulates the entire area, patiently working to relieve that tension by gentle massaging of the external prostate before softly stretching the anus.

It can be a very strong, intimate experience for

lovers to go through and is usually accompanied by a lingam massage.

6. SOAPY MASSAGE

A bathroom can be very stimulating. The soapy massage involves intimate cleaning of a partner in the shower or bathroom where soap is used in place of oil. Not only does this play to the nurturing nature of an intimate relationship, it is also cleans the other for further massaging and sexual interaction. It can likewise serve as a good way to start the day.

7. TANTRIC MASSAGE

These massages involve a list of different techniques derived from elements of yoga, bioenergetics, and sexual therapy. Critically, the receiver is never the giver, it is the job of the receiver to surrender to the sensation of feeling and emotions completely. It is about following feelings of relaxation rather than moving toward an orgasm.

Foreplay serves as the base on which pleasure can be built. All of these, from kissing to massages, work to stimulate, build, and drive desire, resulting in a more intense and pleasurable experience for both parties involved. Within many pieces of literature, there is a notion surrounding sexual energy flowing through the body. Incorporating these foreplay techniques and tips should tap into that sensation of flow—following a natural progression rather than a checklist. Tapping into those natural sensations is a personal journey that can be assisted by these techniques.

3

CLITORAL STIMULATION AND
FEMALE ORGASM

*O*rgasms. Our language lacks the vocabulary to describe the individual experience, but the orgasm has power dissimilar most other body functions. Like other bodily functions, we all experience them differently. No two people have the same orgasm. Some people squirm and sigh, others squirt and scream. Moreover, there are different ways to achieve orgasm—to suggest it is an endzone is missing the larger picture.

Female orgasms are notoriously evasive. Also called "cuming" or "climaxing", having an orgasm is a transcendent experience for both parties. There tend to be weighted expectations placed on the female orgasm by all parties involved. For men, it is seen as a sign of quality while women often feel embarrassed if they cannot climax. In reality, it is not a requirement for "good" sex, nor is it a finish line to hit. Men, you are not failures for not bringing a woman to orgasm. Women, there is nothing wrong with you. Do not lie to men, rather have a conversation about the sex and work collectively toward more pleasure.

Giving your lover an orgasm is one of the great releases in life. Such a philosophical text as the *Kama Sutra* would be remiss to say nothing about them. The first thing it says is fairly straightforward: **women should orgasm first**. It is seen as proof that you understand and respect the needs of your partner. So, what is happening during an orgasm?

There is a slow build before a female orgasm. In direct reaction to prolonged stimulation, the brain is building up a cocktail of dopamine and oxytocin, or the "feel-good" chemicals. This cocktail is designed to prolong the impending ecstasy. It shifts activity from places responsible for anxiety and fear, reinforcing a sense of calm and relaxation. At the same time, the heart rate rises and skin becomes flush as blood rushes around the body. Muscles in the back, pelvis, anus, and vagina all tense rhythmically and involuntarily. Then, all at once, everything releases.

What happens next isn't even up to her. Clawing, squirting, moaning, or screaming: all are on the table. But again, if you read the foreplay section, the orgasm is about a buildup of tension and arousal. It takes time and effort. But this isn't about foreplay. This is about clitoral and vaginal stimulation that leads to orgasm.

Depending on who you talk to, there are between four and eight ways a woman can orgasm. There are many arguments as to how different the experience is for each of these orgasms, but they are all working to stimulate the same set of nerves. In this section, we're going to focus on the four main points of orgasmic stimulation: clitoral, G-spot, A-spot and U-spot.

Clitoral Stimulation

Externally, the clitoris is a single "button" at the top of the vagina. But that's just the tip of the iceberg. Internally, it is a wishbone-shaped nerve the goes around the entire vagina. The single clitoral bulb at the top of the vagina houses over 8,000 nerve endings. Compare this to the penis head's 4,000 nerve endings, and you have yourself a gold medalist in the pleasure Olympics. The most important information: where is the clitoris?

MEDICAL NEWS TODAY

The Vulva

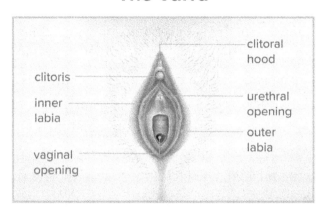

There it is! Notice that it comes with a clitoral hood. This is a variable piece in any sexual experience. Some women prefer you to move the hood and access the clitoris directly. Others cannot take the stimulation and prefer it to be massaged indirectly. Every woman is different, so experiment on the ground. Her body will show you, if you're doing something right. What kind of tools do you have to get her going?

1. SUCK AND NIBBLE

When focusing on the clitoral bulb with your mouth, sucking and nibbling in conjunction with licking are great ways to light her on fire. DO NOT bite. If you're a man, imagine if someone bit your penis, not cool nor pleasurable. DO NOT suck for a prolonged period. Two or three seconds, tops, and then you're off doing something else. Imagine you're gently sucking on a lip. DO NOT punch it into the ground with your tongue.

2. DRAW CIRCLES (ASK)

Leave the alphabet at home. You can do this with your tongue, a single finger, or two fingers. But, as reported by researchers at Indiana University, circles were described as favorites for 3 of 4 women. However, the same study described how women "typically find a pattern and stick with it". 25% of American women aren't doing circles, so asking a woman *how* she likes it is much better than the guessing game that might follow.

3. HINTING

Hinting is when you tease around her clit, making little suggestions and **building tension**. This can be as simple as moving toward, then away, or deliberately playing just beside the clitoris without touching it.

4. PICK A SIDE

Often, a woman has a preferred side for stimulation. Find it, and stick to it.

5. CREATIVE MOTIONS

Paint the fence. Windshield wipers. Figure eight. There are hundreds of fun little motions that can drive a woman crazy.

6. HARMONICA/HUMMINGBIRD

This is an advanced motion. The Harmonica, also known as the Hummingbird, is gently put your lips on the clitoris and humming. This creates a low vibration in the lips and on the clitoris, directly stimulating it. For extra effect, wait until she is already having an orgasm to employ. Again, never bite the clitoris.

7. PENIS MASSAGE

If you're already in the area, why not go for a quick penis massage? Take your erect penis and grind against her clitoris like you're sharpening a knife with a diamond.

8. VIBRATORS/SEX TOYS

Vibrators and sex toys are a great way to directly stimulate the clitoris while doing other things. It's like having a little robot helper in. There are many, many ways to incorporate a plethora of sex toys. For now, a small vibrator resting against the clitoris will free you to hit other erogenous zones and, maybe, even add to your own pleasure.

U-Spot

This is also outside of the vagina—the **urethra**. Recently defined and not mentioned in the *Kama Sutra*, but worth mentioning here, the U-spot is the skin on the upper part of the vagina. Many people suspect it is a part of the unlying clitoral structure, but most important is the stimulation it provides.

You can stimulate the U-spot using the same tools mentioned for the clitoris—any combination of pressure, temperature, and speed will produce different results. Many people discover its existence when the partner rubs their penis up and down the length of the vagina. Find what works and go with it!

G-Spot

The fabled G-spot is the most accessible pleasure point within the vagina, located between 2-3" (5-8 cm) on the roof. The skin there is typically distinct from the other parts of the canal, sporting a ribbed texture rather than the smooth surrounding it.

It is not a magical button that lets women climax on command. As all other erogenous spots, it is important that you massage it, keeping note as to how she reacts to different pressures and motions. Again, every woman is different. Experimentation is always the route to orgasm.

Fortunately, there is also an entire industry dedicated to experimentation. If you have not already invested in a sex toy, there are many specifically curved to stimulate and pleasure the G-spot.

A-Spot

This is the second interior pleasure point of the vagina. This spot was only described medically in the 1990s, so it is relatively unknown to a majority of the population.

If you think of the vaginal canal as a tunnel, the G-spot is on one end with the A-Spot on the other. The A-spot is a different experience stimulated by deeper penetration rather than the shallow action of the G-spot.

This spot is either reached with the penis, the fingers, or a sex toy—it requires deep penetration and relaxation. Thankfully, it does not suffer from post-orgasm sensitivity like the clitoris does, making it the ideal candidate for delivering multiple, back to back orgasms. However, 75% of women cannot experience an orgasm from penetration alone; the A-spot is often an afterthought rather than a sought out local. But if she's asking to go deeper, this is what she's asking you to hit.

Notes on Penetration Techniques

1. FINGERING AND THE COME HITHER

Penetrating a woman with your fingers is one of the easiest ways to get her stimulated and climaxing. A man's stamina is often less than the amount of time she needs; fingering is the best way to close that gap.

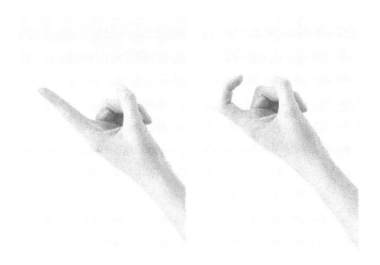

Of these methods, the "come hither" motion is the best way to stimulate an orgasm. It directly stimulates the G-spot.

Fingering does not always need to mimic the in and out of the penis. Resting the fingers inside the vagina, gently perusing around the edges, and variable motions are all great ways to get her going in fun, easy ways.

2. PENIS PENETRATION

The penis is not a piston, and a man is not a giant dildo with some extra bits. When the penis is inside the vagina, a way to get a woman closer to climax is to hit these spots consistently. There are specific positions described in the *Kama Sutra* that will be reviewed later, but for now, understanding these anatomic structures is key to producing a female orgasm.

Things Preventing Climax

Sometimes, an inability to climax has nothing to do with the sexual partner or act itself.

1. Anxiety: Anxiety during sex is very common for all parties involved. The best way to address this during safe sex is, almost in a meditative fashion, focus on the pleasure. What does it feel like? In the same way you might focus on your breath, focus on the sensations of the body.

2. Not Tensing Muscles: The muscles need to be strong enough to involuntarily tense. If you aren't climaxing, it may be a good idea

to manually clench your kegel muscles and botox.

3. Lubrication: Sex is dirty. Make sure it is also slippery. Even if this is achieved naturally, there is never harm in adding some lube to the mix.

4. Self-Restriction: Afraid to lose control, make noise or communicate? Focusing on these three common forms of self restriction not only increases anxiety, it also prevents your natural expression of ecstasy. For men, be sure to encourage this behavior through prompts and assurances. If this becomes too difficult or scary to do, it may be a good idea to speak to a sex therapist.

5. Medication: Many forms of medication can affect the ability for a woman to climax at all. Be sure to research your specific brand to see if this is a side effect. If it is, speak to a doctor about alternatives or solutions.

One of the most searched sexual questions on Google is "how to give a woman an orgasm". But the answer isn't in a cheap magazine that needs to sell another copy the next week. The answer comes from human anatomy and the many different cultural experiences of pleasure over the course of human existence. Good on you for doing your research. That already puts you ahead of the pack! But stimulation of human genitals doesn't stop with foreplay and the clitoris. In the next chapter, we're taking a look at oral sex.

4

ORAL SEX

We all have the same parts. The penis and the clitoris stem from the same nerve endings before a baby is gendered, the prostate and the G-spot as well. More obviously, men and women share a mouth: a well-lubricated, pleasure machine. There is something beyond the sensations you can feel through the lips alone, the intimacy and passion that can be conveyed through a kiss: oral sex.

Oral sex is not uniquely human, but language is. Thousands of generations of blow job bestowing and mons munchin' has brought us to a unique moment in time. It is possible to learn, share and experiment with new ideas together. There are many things that humanity has learned: this chapter will review blow jobs, going down on a woman, and some of the best positions to try.

Intro to Blow Job

More than anything, a blow job is about the extra bells and whistles you bring to it. Enthusiasm, suction, noise, lubrication, hand usage, and many more factors contribute to the quality of a blow job. What is important is that you make it yours! A signature move in your arsenal of sex moves. First though, lets better understand what makes up the male penis.

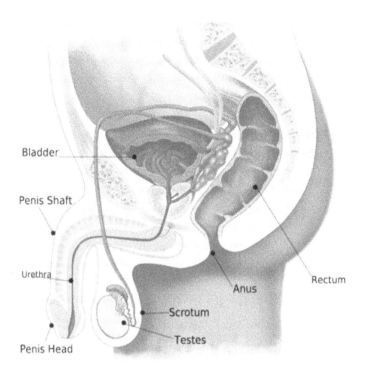

Bladder

Penis Shaft

Urethra

Penis Head

Rectum

Anus

Scrotum

Testes

Penises come in all different sizes, but the shape is relatively consistent. As shown above, there are between three and four main areas for stimulation: the head, the shaft, the scrotum, and the foreskin (optional).

Most penises are well kept and groomed. Certain realities must be understood before going into a blow job. The first is how many men masturbate. This is something to talk about with the man, but it is not uncommon for a man to sprint through a masturbation to get to the climax. It is often more of a well-lubricated milking. They may not feel as though they have time, do it in secrecy, and don't take the time to explore themselves thoroughly. Your job, as the person bestowing the blow job, is to show him the error of his ways. There are a few things to consider first.

To Avoid

There are a few things to keep in mind, but the biggest killer of any blow job is the involvement of teeth. Teeth scraping down the side of the penis is not comfortable or pleasurable for the man and is often painful. Be careful and don't stress. Go only as far as you feel comfortable going.

Remember that hygiene comes before all. If a penis is not well kept, that is a free pass to evacuate. If a penis smells bad, has any sort of suspicious bumps or boils, do not put your mouth near it.

Things He Wants You to Know

Remember that the head of the penis and clitoris are very, very similar. One of the more important things shared between the two of them is their sensitivity after an orgasm. As a man builds closer and closer to orgasm, the head of his penis is becoming more and more sensitive. After an orgasm, he is extremely sensitive. Do not be surprised if he tries to keep you from doing anything after he cums. It is a natural reaction to intense and sudden sensitivity.

By the same token, there is an opportunity to increase pleasure. Light touch can be extremely stimulating. With the penis out of the mouth, a light lick, kiss, or gentle rub can be a great way to tease every ounce of pleasure from a blow job.

Many seemingly little things can change the feel of a blow job. The location of the blow job can be a major factor. Switching it up from the bedroom to another place, simply from lying down to standing up, or to any of the upcoming positions are great ways to add a spark to a blow job. Further, eye contact, prostate probing, and sloppiness are all great factors to consider when giving a blow job.

Hands are an important piece of the puzzle. If your hands are not touching the penis, there are many other great areas to put them. Grabbing his butt, under his thighs and in the crevice of his knees are all great locations. The goal is to communicate enthusiasm.

The cherry on top of every blow job is the creativity of it! Location and positioning can be changed easily, but what else? Temperature, maybe? A blow job with ice cubes in your mouth? The more creative and enthusiastic, the better it comes off!

Lastly, more than anything, he hopes you enjoy yourself as well. Remember that there isn't a right way to give a blow job, that you're building a pleasure bar. Do as you like and experiment.

Spit or Swallow

This question is a source of tension for many people giving blow jobs. Some people don't like the taste of semen or have negatively associated with it while others enjoy it. Finding an enjoyable way to work with the semen after a man climaxes is up to the person giving the blow job.

Swallowing semen is not and should not be considered a gross act, nor is it out of the norm. If you feel uncomfortable with the taste, but still want to swallow, time the motion so that the man orgasms while the head of his penis is toward the back of your throat.

If you prefer neither of these options, you're more than welcome to take the penis out of your mouth and stroke it at a pace consistent with the mouth until he cums. Be careful to consider cleanup afterward!

With regard to kissing afterward, it is up to the individuals involved. Some men don't want to taste their own cum while others don't mind. A good way to clean the cum off of your lips is to kiss his body as you move from his penis toward his mouth.

Inspirations

1. Regular Blow Job Positions
2. Kneeling: The woman kneels in front of the standing man
3. Relaxed: Both the woman and man are lying down
4. Face Fuck Position: With the woman lying down, the man straddles her as she grips his hips
5. Raised Blow Job Positions
6. Bosses Chair: With the man sitting back in a chair, the woman sits on her knees.
7. Cinema position: Sitting side by side, the woman bends over
8. Doctor's Office: With the man lying down

on a reclined sofa and the woman kneeling to the side

9. Creative Blow Job Positions

10. The 69: Facing opposite direction, one on top of the other, the two provide simultaneous fellatio

11. The Jack Hammer: With the man standing, the woman positions herself directly under him

12. Thigh Pillow: Similar to the 69, but both parties are on the side rather than on top of one another

Intro to Going Down

Going down on a woman is one of the unique pleasures in life. It is similar to a blow job for men, but held in higher regard because most men cannot climax without it. Do not misunderstand. An ability to go down on a woman is what separates the boys from the men (or girls from the women). If you ever feel uncomfortable about questions of stamina or length, being able to rock a woman's world before sex even begins is the easiest way to satisfy her.

Do...

All of the previous ideas of making a woman

comfortable apply here, maybe even more so. Before you even get near the vagina, make sure you've kissed every inch of her body. This is also a good way to probe if she's clean. Don't dive in and regret it later. But when she comes back clean, the name of the game is suspense and tension. Play with that before you play with anything else. Rubbing, touching, biting, and teasing are all prerequisites. Be sure it doesn't feel like a checklist. Once she's begging you to go down, the real work begins.

1. CONFIDENCE

Remember, the first rule of any sexual interaction is to make the other person feel confident. In this situation, that means quelling some fears women have. Tell her she tastes good when she does, that you're excited to go down, and show some enthusiasm! You should have more than a few tricks up your sleeve after this chapter.

2. HIT OTHER PARTS OF THE VAGINA

The clitoris is a fantastic place to deliver some high-quality pleasure, but don't forget about the other parts of her body! "Labia, labia, vulva" is a great motto as you work your way in. Don't be afraid to get down and dirty. You're already there, so commit and don't look back!

3. BUT WHEN YOU DO...

Figure out how she likes it. As mentioned in the foreplay chapter, women tend to have a specific motion they enjoy more than others. If you haven't already, ask her. If you don't ask her, the best bet is a circular motion, but experiment. Throw her body a curveball and see how she reacts.

4. CHANGE THE CLOCK

You're going to want to orient yourself based on P.S.T: pressure, sucking, and temperature. Get creative with how you implement these into the experience. How are you going to apply pressure? Nose, lips, tongue, chin, fingers? Maybe a sex toy? These are completely up to you. Just make sure the area is properly lubricated. Sucking is kryptonite. Use it wisely. Do not suck for too long. One one-thousand, two one-thousand, and you're off of there. Temperature control can be a cherry on top. Some light blowing can cool down the saliva while hot

ORAL SEX | 55

breath tells her you're into it. These three are the knobs to calibrate. Find a spot that she likes, then hold it. Keep it consistent until she cums.

Don't...

There are a lot of nerve endings down there. Everywhere you turn, there are nerves slowly building toward a climax. There are more than a few things that can go wrong.

1. SWITCHING IT UP AT THE FINISH LINE

You've just run a race. You're almost to the finish line. Her body is screaming at you. She may even be screaming at you. Do not randomly turn left just before you get to the finish line. Keep it consistent. Give her the first orgasm. If she says, "don't stop", don't stop. If you want to try another move later, that's a great time to experiment.

2. LOOK

There seems to be some debate on this. When women make eye contact while giving a blow job, it can be a massive turnon for a guy. When guys do it to women, it tends to have the opposite effect. The amount of focus and willpower it takes for a woman to climax isn't worth distracting from and risking in the name of a little eye contact (unless blatantly instructed otherwise).

3. TEETH = BAD

For men, how would you feel if a girl bit your penis? Multiply that by two, and that's about the response you could expect if you bite a woman's clitoris. If you need to bite anywhere, bite her inner thigh.

4. BLATANTLY INSTRUCTED OTHERWISE

Again, women are all different. What works for one may not work at all for another. Make sure you're working based on her feedback, physical or verbal, rather than following a strategy guide written by Men's Weekly. Listen to what she says!

5. SLOPPY JOE

The vagina is not a sandwich. Do not jump down and start aggressively munching. Make sure it is a controlled descent the entire way, matching her rhythm and listening to her body.

Things She Wants You to Know

1. IT ISN'T AN EXCHANGE

Many women believe oral sex to be more intimate than normal sex. Not only is it often a critical piece to get her to climax, but it is also something she values very highly. So don't think it's a tit for tat, "you do me then I'll do" kind of setup. Do it because it will make her feel good, harboring an ulterior motive is a real mood killer.

2. STAY INVOLVED ELSEWHERE

When you're going down, you've become World War 1 Germany—two fronts! While your mouth and maybe a few fingers are operating down below, your other hand needs to be hitting other areas of interest. Rubbing and grabbing the nipples is highly appreciated; some women also enjoy fingers in their mouths. Others enjoy a probing finger in or around the anus. The important thing is to keep her going on multiple fronts!

3. ENTHUSIASM IS KEY!

The same advice applies to blowjobs, correct? Enjoy yourself down there! It's a little adventure to quickly figure out what makes her feel good, maybe even so much that she orgasms. Great creative, too! Add some ice cubes, a vibrator, or stimulate the G-Spot at the same time. The clam is your oyster!

Inspirations

1. *The Faceplant:* The man lies on his back, has the woman hovering above him as he caresses her while eating her out
2. *The Sidecar*: Start lying side by side, face to face. Then slide down, kissing her until you reach the vagina.
3. *The Standing 69*: Start in a classic 69 position, then slowly start getting up, holding her in place as you lift off the bed. Make sure once you do, she is facing the bed should she fall!
4. *Cliff Hanger*: The woman lies at the edge of the bed, legs draped over the man kneeling on the ground in front of her
5. *Doggie*: The woman sits on all fours in front of the man, who eats her from behind. A good position for eating booty as well!

5

BEGINNER SEX POSITIONS IN THE KAMA SUTRA

*S*ex in the *Kama Sutra* is contained within 64 positions for intercourse, all perfected and passed down from generation to generation. This section contains some of the easiest positions to get started with, as well as some more modern takes on the positions of old.

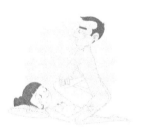

1. THE BANDOLEER

The woman begins by lying on her back cushion under her head. From there, she lifts both legs to her chest while the man kneels in front of her. She rests her feet on his chest and her hips on his thighs. He puts his forearms across her legs as he penetrates her.

From there, she can grab his hips and lower thighs, controlling the thrusting. The weight of the woman and man should counterbalance, resulting in a relaxing position with deeper penetration.

A pillow under the man's legs could help stabilize the whole position if you're having trouble balancing.

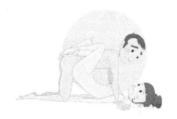

2. THE GRIP

Begin with the woman lying down in a missionary position. The man approaches for above and enters missionary style. From there, he lifts up on all fours while the woman wraps her legs around his waist, keeping the penis inside of her.

This position allows the woman to thrust and hump with the penis, using her legs and hips. As a tip, it is a good idea to lock your feet on the man's lower back to allow for better control and stability.

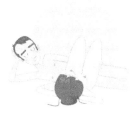

3. AFTERNOON DELIGHT

The man and woman lay perpendicular to one another. The man, on his side, enters the woman, who is draping her legs around his hips. This allows easy, tight penetration. The woman swivels her hips while the man is free to thrust, assisted by the woman's legs should she choose.

This position is great because it liberates three hands to do other things or simply enjoy the casual afternoon delight. It is also a perfect cool-down position for long sex sessions in a large bed.

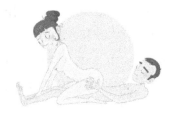

4. THE RIDER

A little more relaxed but still very similar to reverse cowgirl, the Rider incorporates the woman's hands as critical support. The man lays flat while the woman straddles him, facing his feet. Her knees are on the surface parallel with his legs. As she takes the penis into her vagina, she leans forward and places her hands on his shins.

This is great for a woman who wants to control the penetration while providing a great view for the man. It may be a good idea to cover the feet with a sheet or blanket if the woman is made uncomfortable by them.

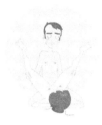

5. THE EAGLE

The woman lays down flat with the man between her legs. The man lifts the hips and the legs gently, gripping above the knee, as far as the ankles depending on flexibility. He slips into her while raising her hips and allowing for deeper penetration.

A small pillow or crumpled blanket helps enormously with the physical burden of this position. Placing it just under the woman's hips allows more comfort with the same depth of penetration.

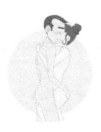

6. THE VISITOR

While standing at an equal height, the man and woman face each other. The man rubs his penis against her vulva, stimulating and gently probing into her.

Any disparity in height will throw this position into chaos. The height factor can be overcome through heels, stairs, or creativity.

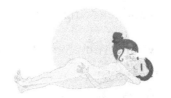

7. THE SLIDE

With the man lying flat, the woman lays on top of him. She crosses her arms behind the man's neck, allowing him to rest his nape on her forearms. Her feet are press against the inside of the ankles. Using her toes and forearms as leverage and with her legs close together, she slides up and down on his penis. The man grips the hips, but ultimately enjoys the ride.

This makes for an intimate experience delivered by the woman. The man is relatively inactive but can supplement the affection with kisses and handiness.

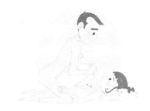

8. THE TOMINAGI

This position is very similar to the Bandoleer with one critical difference. Again, the woman is on her back with the feet resting on the chest of the man. The man, after entering her, should place the weight of his upper body on the knees of the woman, holding them steady rather than letting her move them freely.

This shifts the power of the position to the man, enabling a deeper penetration with consistency. The Tominagi is a great position for less endowed men and/or men who like to take control.

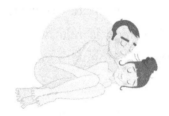

9. THE CURLED ANGEL

Born of a big spoon-little spoon dynamic, the man and the woman are in a cuddling position. The man lowers himself to be inline with the woman's opening, thrusting from behind as she relaxes with her knees held to her chest.

This is a great position for a light, tired or lazy

evening of loving. This position is also good for pregnant women. The woman only needs to gently lower her knees to accommodate a bump.

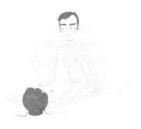

10. THE CROSS

The woman is spread out, one leg lying extended and flat. The man straddles the extended leg while lifting the other, bent at the knee and resting on his chest. He enters her softly and thrusts using pelvic muscles rather than leaning over, keeping the knee bent at a 90-degree angle.

This position shines when the woman is tired or as a transitional position. It is also a great way to specifically target the G-spot with his penis.

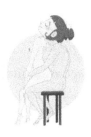

11. THE PERCH

A stool or chair is needed for this position. While a man is sitting down, a woman approaches. She turns her back to him and rests teasingly on his penis, working it in slowly. The woman is in complete control of her motion: Circling, bouncing, or humping are all options. This position is hands-free, allowing for her to grab his legs or neck and him to play with her clitoris or breasts.

This position is ideal for a tired man or a pregnant woman.

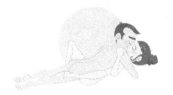

12. THE TOAD

It begins with a missionary. The woman lies on her back with her legs open while the man lays on top of her. With his legs extended behind him, he wraps his arms around her caressingly. She, likewise, wraps her legs around his torso. She controls the pressure and force of his pelvic motion by pushing on his buttocks with her legs.

This is a lovemaking position; a romantic setting is highly recommended, as well as a slower, intimate pace.

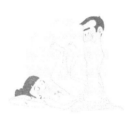

13. THE HERO

With the woman lying on her back, she brings her knees to her chest with her feet pointing up. From there, the man kneels. He pushes back on the inside of her knees, pulling her hips up, and slides his thighs under her hips for support. Finally, he inserts the penis while keeping pressure on the inside of the knees and support under the hips.

This position is a more difficult one but great for deeper penetration. It is a starting point for couples who are looking to begin more difficult positions.

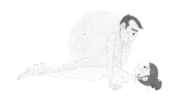

14. THE CLASSIC

Very similar to the missionary position with one slight alteration. Rather than the woman lying flat on the surface, there is a small pillow or cushion under her bottom. The slight tilt of the pelvis allows the penis and vaginal canals to align, enabling deeper and more seamless penetration than a typical missionary style.

This can be a great starting position if the penis is

the first thing to enter the vagina, or if the woman is a little dry.

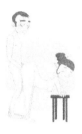

15. THE FAN

The woman bends over to lean on a supportive structure, crossing her arms and putting pressure on her elbows as she does so. The man then enters from behind, controlling the depth and pressure of the penetration by holding the top of her thighs.

This is another position where the height disparity is an important factor to be considered. The larger the disparity, the more difficult the position will be to achieve satisfaction. A few other factors to consider are the width, angle, and flexibility of the woman's legs. Regardless, this position is great for anal sex!

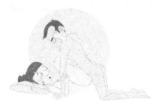

16. THE SNAIL

With the woman on her back already, she pulls her knees to her chest. The man kneels in front of her and enters. With him inside, the woman lifts her legs and rests them on his shoulders as the man leans forward, placing both arms on either side of her as support.

For added comfort and depth, a pillow to support the head and neck of the woman is a great addition. The penetration with this position is very deep, making if great for hitting the A-spot. It is a good idea not to go too fast while thrusting.

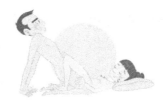

17. THE SLIP

Here, the man first kneels back with the woman lying in front of him, flat on her back. The man leans back, placing his arms behind to support himself. The woman places her legs comfortably around the man's hips, inching her own hips toward him to ease penetration.

As a relatively easy, highly penetrative position, this is a great one to incorporate. However, it is better to transition into another similar position rather than beginning with. The man simply needs to lean back while the woman holds on and adjusts.

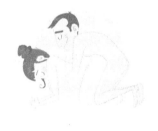

18. THE HOUND

This one's very similar to doggy style but differs in structural support. Rather than being on all fours, the woman supports herself using her forearms, creating an arched back. He then enters from behind, hands free and able to caress her simultaneously.

Be sure to do this on a comfortable surface like a bed or couch, as much of the two peoples' weights will be concentrated on the woman's forearms!

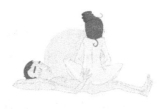

19. THE SHIP

While the man is lying flat on his back, the woman sits on top of him. Rather than sitting toward or away from him, she sits perpendicular to his pelvis, forming a cross with their pelvic bones. She has complete control of the motion, penetration, and speed of the sex.

This is more exhaustive for the woman than the man, but it is still a very simple change to a common position that focuses on comfort. The man is hands free and able to rub and caress the woman. For increased penetration, remove the pillow from behind the head and place it under the hips.

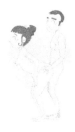

20. FROM BEHIND

The woman, facing a wall, leans against it while the man enters her from behind. He is in control of the thrusts and motion throughout the position.

It is important to again consider height disparity. To compensate, the woman can lean forward and lift her heels while the man can squat and spread his legs. This is a great position for unorthodox locations or showers.

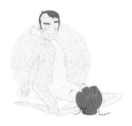

21. SPLITTING BAMBOO

The woman lays on her back, draping one leg over the man's shoulder with the other extended behind him. The man straddles the extended leg at the thigh, holding onto the elevated leg for balance and control.

The woman is free to touch and caress either herself or the man while the man maintains control of the body. This form is a relatively easy position to transition into from a missionary position, though it is best when begun from a position that already straddles the leg.

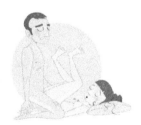

22. THE CANDLE

The woman lies on her back, pillows below her hips and her head, pushing her into a more curled position. With her legs up, the weight of which are over her chest, the man kneels and positions his legs on either side of her hips. He enters her, hands-free, for a deep penetration.

The key to this move is the position of the woman's body; the concave arch of the body allows greater depth and stimulation. All hands are free in this position, so if the pillow is not enough, lifting up on the woman's hips will help create that concave angle needed.

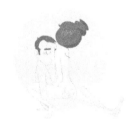

23. THE BASKET

While the man stretches out one leg, the other is

bent at the knee, creating a stable and controlled base. The woman then sits on his lap, inserting his penis. While she is in control of much of the movement, he can control and lift her using his free hands.

This position is the perfect position for sex while simultaneously stimulating the nipples. The question of the woman's legs is up to her. Wrapping them around the man will result in less control while having them fixed on the ground will increase control.

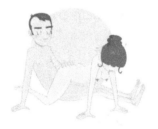

24. THE GALLEY

With his legs extended in front of him, the man leans to the side and puts his weight on one arm. The woman sits on top of him, straddling his hips and taking in the penis. From there, she leans to the side and, using her arms to support her, aligns herself with the man's structure.

This position gives the woman control of the motion and penetration. The man also has one hand free, allowing him to fondle the clitoris or bottom.

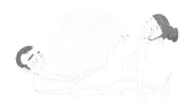

25. THE CLIP

The man lies back in bed, closing his legs and allowing room for the woman to comfortably straddle him. The woman gets on top, taking in the penis. She then leans back and focuses the weight on her arms, grinding.

This position is a great view for the man, but can be exhausting for a prolonged period for the woman. This move is a great transitional move in between a cowgirl or another female-mounted position.

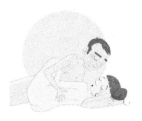

26. THE WHISPER

With the woman lying on her back, she wraps her legs around the man as he enters her. The man then lays on his side or props himself up with his forearm.

This is a fantastic transitional position, that retains a sense of intimacy and mobility while allowing for mutual control. The woman is free to hump and pull the man into her with her legs while he can control the speed and tempo of the sex.

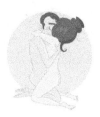

27. THE KNEEL

The impassioned position starts with both partners in a kneeling position. The woman puts either of her legs to the side of one of the man's, allowing him to penetrate her. This allows both parties to wrap their arms around each other.

If there is a significant height difference between the man and the woman, there are a few ways to address it. If the man is shorter, he can put a pillow under the straddled knee. However, if the woman is shorter, it is best that the man lifts her up onto the leg.

28. THE SPHINX

The woman, lying on her stomach, lifts her chest and places the weight on her forearms. She then stretches one leg out behind, the other tucked forward. The man then lays on top of her, entering from behind while holding his body up with his arms.

This position can be very tiring for the man but does a great job of positioning the woman in a perfect spot for a G-spot-driven climax.

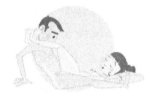

29. THE DECK CHAIR

Sitting with his legs stretched forward, the man leans back on his hands. The woman, lying in between his legs with a pillow behind her head, raises her own legs and places them on his shoulders. The man inserts himself.

While the man has limited ability to thrust, the woman can rotate and grind on the penis, as well as move back and forth. Her free hands act as leverage points, further enabling her control. This position is good for deep, slower penetration in a relaxed environment.

30. THE DOUBLE DECKER

While the man is on his back. The woman, lying in the same direction with her back on his chest, lays on top of him. He holds her hips while she places her elbows down, grounding them both to the surface. Her feet are placed either on the knees, shins, or ankles of the man.

This is a position designed for transitioning. A great way to accentuate this position is for the man to place one of his hands on another erogenous zone— same for her!

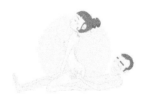

31. THE REVERSE COWGIRL

The man starts lying on his back. The woman straddles over him, facing his feet, and slides down the penis. The woman has complete discretion over the motion, speed, and depth.

This move is such a classic, providing a stimulating view for the man and full control for the woman.

32. THE LOTUS BLOSSOM

The man, sitting cross legged, invites the woman to sit on his lap. The woman puts her legs behind him, lowers herself onto his penis, then wraps her legs and arms around him. The two face each other.

This position is great for couples who want an easier, intimate position with equal control. Both have open hands with the bonus of being face to face with one another.

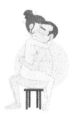

33. THE AMAZON

This position requires a chair, preferably open back, that isn't too high. The man should begin by sitting in the chair. The woman then sits on his lap, inserting him into her. Using her feet to push off the ground, she bounces up and down.

This position requires a very specific prop, as well as some strength on behalf of both parties. An easy way to improve it is simply by adjusting the bend of the man's knees. It is also a fantastic transition between standing and lying positions.

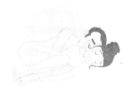

34. THE CLOSE UP

The man and woman both lie together in a spooning position. Their legs are intertwined, pulled up toward the chest of the woman. Facing away from the man, she pushes her hips into his hips as he inserts himself.

This is a soothing, gentle and intimate position that is more designed to caress each other in conjunction with stimulation.

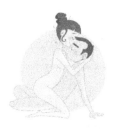

35. THE ROCKING HORSE

The man begins by sitting with his legs crossed, arms behind him to support the weight of his torso. The woman then soothingly straddles him, leaning on his body and holding him as she puts him inside of her. Rather than bouncing up and down like other mounted positions, the woman rocks back and forth, grinding up and down on the man.

This position can be extremely intimate, keeping the control with the woman regarding speed and penetration. However, the key is to resist the temptation to thrust or bounce. Be sure to vary the speed of the grinding, but this position is not suitable for fast bouncing or thrusting.

36. THE SUPER EIGHT

While the woman lies straight on her back with raised hips, the man lies between her legs. Supporting himself by raising his arms, he inserts himself. Both the man and the woman can move in conjunction with one another, allowing for very rhythmic sex.

This position can become tiring for the man, specifically in the arms. However, it is a great move for sex while listening to music.

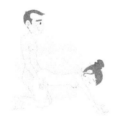

37. DOGGY STYLE

This classic position begins with the woman on all fours. The man comes from behind, entering her from behind. The man is in control of this position, though the woman can press back into him.

While both the woman's hands are occupied, the

man has two free hands. One of these can reach around and stimulate an erogenous zone, or use them to hold onto the hips of the woman. This is a good finishing position.

38. THE NIRVANA

This position works best with a bedpost or some structure physically above the woman for her to grab onto. She lays flat with her legs together, gripping the bedpost above. The man lays with her legs between his, keeping them together with the placement of his knees. He then enters her slowly while her legs remain shut.

This position is also commonly used in sex with restraints or bondage. The position can be improved by the man setting one arm behind the woman's head and the other with her hand on the bedpost.

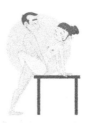

39. THE PADLOCK

With the woman sitting on a higher piece of furniture or countertop, she leans back onto her arms and opens her legs. Standing directly in front of her, she wraps her legs around him at the waist, pulling him toward her as he enters her.

The man should adjust the angle he is standing based on the height of the piece of furniture. For deeper penetration, the woman should keep her hips as close to the edge as possible.

40. THE ROCK N' ROLLER (BEGINNER)

A woman on her back with a pillow below her head lifts her legs in the air. She does so as if she is rolling onto her shoulders. The man then straddles her raised hips, keeping them off the ground by holding them elevated on his thighs. From here, he enters her with his head bent over between her legs or shins. Together, the two rock back and forth together.

This position is good for deep penetration, allowing for very intimate sex. A great tip for this position is to place a pillow under the legs of the man to push him forward.

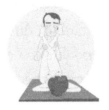

41. THE CROSSED KEY

The woman lies on her back toward the edge of the bed, raising her legs. The man crosses them at the ankles, placing them on the shoulder or holding them in front of him. With the legs crossed and straight (or slightly bent), the man penetrates her while holding onto the legs.

This is an easy sex position that allows deeper penetration. The woman's hands are free to caress herself. This position is great if there are other people involved or if the location is a character in the experience.

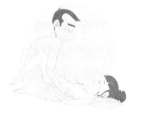

42. THE WIDE OPEN

The complete opposite of The Crossed Key—the wide open begins with the woman lying down, pillow supporting her head. The man kneels under her, raising her hips onto his legs as he enters her. The woman is free to rotate her hips around while the man can thrust gently.

This is a more delicate position. Neither person has much leverage. This makes it a great position for relaxing and calming the mood.

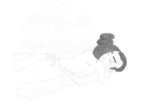

43. THE PEG

This is very similar to the slide but changes to accommodate a well-endowed man. The man's leg spread out, stretched and parted. The woman rest on his chest, arms draped around the man's neck with her feet now on the outside of his ankles. As the penis enters her, she rubs up and down with closed legs, creating tightness while both parties soothe each other with their bodies.

6

ADVANCED KAMA SUTRA POSITIONS
(TIPS AND TRICKS)

*A*ll of these require a certain amount of strength, balance, flexibility, and stamina to achieve. But if you're trying to bring your sexual antics to the next level, this is that level! These positions are not only fun and challenging to achieve, they are great ways to achieve new and exciting orgasm. While many of these have been sourced directly from the *Kama Sutra*, there are also a few modern and equally challenging techniques. It goes without saying, be careful and enjoy yourselves!

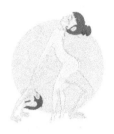

1. THE BRIDGE

The bridge is for extremely strong and flexible men. The man arches his back and places his hands on the floor such that his head is upside-down facing the ground. Meanwhile, he extends his hips and allows the woman to sit and insert his penis from atop his hips. The exertion produces a wild, animalistic orgasm within the man while the woman, using her feet, is free to move up and down on him.

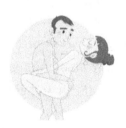

2. THE CLASP

With the man standing, she straddles his waist and wraps her legs around his waist as he supports her hips and back. This is ideal for any location but can be improved if the woman has a wall or support structure to lean against.

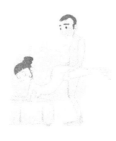

3. THE PLOUGH

With the woman places at the edge of the bed, legs hanging off, the man positions himself between her legs. He lifts her hips and thighs, allowing for penetration, while she supports herself on her elbows. For even more support, the woman can lock her legs into the man's back.

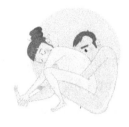

4. THE SEATED BALL

A more unorthodox position, the woman crouches onto the man's lap. She controls the penetration throughout the position by using her heels to rock back and forth on the man. The man holds onto the woman from behind, thrusting into her while keeping his core tight.

5. THE GLOWING JUNIPER

The woman lies on her back with her legs bent apart. The man sits, facing her, with his legs to either side of her. He then lifts her onto him, penetrating and holding her. This is a very easy position for the woman but requires some flexibility on the part of the man.

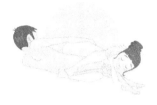

6. THE PEG

With the man on his side, the woman curls up into a ball with her head toward his feet. She wraps her legs around his, her arms around her legs, while he enters her almost upside down. This can be difficult to initiate but can be a great transition from reverse cowgirl!

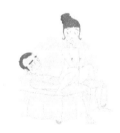

7. THE CROUCHING TIGER

While the man hangs his legs off the bed, bottom toward the edge, the woman squats over him with her feet to either side of his hips. She's facing the other direction but in complete control of the depth and pace of the penetration. This position, while easy and great for the man, requires a good amount of strength from the woman. There is also a high risk of falling off the bed, so be careful!

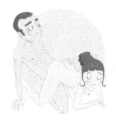

8. THE HINGE

The man, kneeling behind the woman, leans back and begins supporting himself with one arm. The woman kneels in front of him and, using the support of her elbows, thrusts back into him.

9. THE BALANCING ACT

The man begins by lying on his back with his legs apart. The woman then sits between his thighs, facing away from him. She curls her body up into a ball while the man works to support her. While keeping her steady, he can lift and penetrate her as she caresses him or herself.

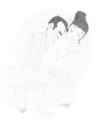

10. THE FROG

The man starts by sitting on the edge of the bed, feet on the floor. The woman crouches on his lap, legs spread open. From that stance, she bounces up and down on his penis, controlling depth and frequency of penetration, leaning on his thighs for support.

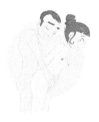

11. THE COLUMN

With their arms intertwined, the man and woman stand together. The man penetrates her from behind. The difficulty with this position comes with the combination of balance and motion. The two need to focus on counterbalancing the thrusts by holding onto one another.

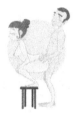

12. THE CHALLENGE

Aptly named, the challenge requires a chair or stool. The woman crouches on the stool while the man enters her from behind, firmly grasping her waist to keep her from toppling over as he thrusts. Be sure to pick a stable chair or stool of appropriate height. If it has a back, the woman should hold onto it with her hands.

13. THE KNEELING WHEELBARROW

Kneeling with one leg stretched out at the hip, the woman leans on the opposite elbow (i.e., right elbow, left leg). Her partner kneels behind her, supporting the weight of her leg by holding her hips as he enters her. Best done when the woman locks her leg while the man supports it, allowing it to last longer.

14. THE STANDING WHEELBARROW

With the woman on all fours, resting her elbows on a pillow or soft surface, the man enters from behind. Once inside, the man slowly lifts her off the ground, holding her ankles, all while maintaining the union of penis and vagina.

Be sure to lift from the ankles, but keep the ankles under the hips! Do not let them extend beyond the weight of the woman's torso.

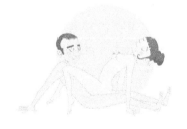

15. THE SPIDER

The man, with outstretched legs and arms behind him, leans back. The woman sits on top of him, facing him, with her legs behind him and arms betwixt his legs. From there, she begins to rock back and forth. This is a great position that gives both parties limited control. Tossing the head back helps bring you into the position even more!

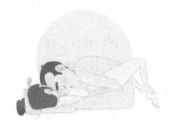

16. THE FOLD

The woman lies on her back with her hips raised by an aptly placed pillow. The man, with legs stretched out to either side of the woman, enters her. The woman's legs are either falling behind him or locked while he is able to touch, lick and caress her body.

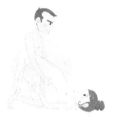

17. THE DOLPHIN

With the woman lying on her back, the man situates himself between her legs. Lifting from the waist or bottom, he puts all of her weight on her head or shoulders. From there, he penetrates her, maintaining the same height throughout the move. While this is easy enough to do, it is harder to maintain over a long period! If the arm is long enough, the man can situate his forearms under the woman's thighs, relieving strain.

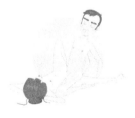

18. THE STAR

As the woman lies on her back, she stretches one leg out while bending the other at the knee. The man slides in between her legs, pushing one of his legs—extended—under her hips and along the side of her back. He then leans back on his arms and penetrates her. This is a great position for G-spot stimulation. The woman has free hands as well!

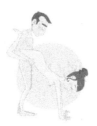

19. THE INDIAN HANDSTAND

The man stands while the woman does a handstand or headstand. The man enters her, allowing her to lean back on him while helping her balance using his hands. This is a difficult one that can be made easier if the woman digs her heels into the back of the man, providing more stability. The man can also lift up on the woman, offering light relief to her arms.

20. ASCENT TO DESIRE

The man, standing with his knees slightly bent, faces the standing woman. He then lifts her off the ground, grabbing her bottom or upper thigh, and penetrates her. The woman wraps her legs around his waist, arms around his neck.

This is also made easier if there is a table, bed or small chair behind the man for the woman to lightly place her feet. It is also possible to begin penetration in a sitting position, then switch to a standing one.

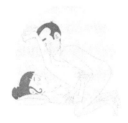

21. THE ROCK N' ROLLER (ADVANCED)

While the woman begins by lying on her back with a pillow behind her head, she rocks her legs back as if to do a backward roll. The man kneels in front of her, catches her mid-roll, and enters her while keeping the hips elevated. The woman then rocks back and forth as the man thrusts.

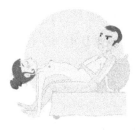

22. THE BACKWARD SLIDE

With a cushion supporting his back, the man sits at the edge of the bed with his legs hanging off. The woman straddles him, bending her knees so that they are level with his shoulders. After inserting him, she leans back and places her hands on either the ground or his feet/ankles.

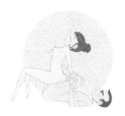

23. THE APE

As the man lays on his back, he brings his knees to his chest. The woman, facing away from him, sits on the backside of his thighs and inserts his penis. With his feet on her back, the woman uses her feet to balance and control the depth of penetration and speed of movement. For added support, it might be a good idea to hold each others' wrists!

24. THE RECLINING LOTUS

The woman begins by lying on her back with legs crossed. As the man lays on top of her, she should place her feet into the grooves of his hips. The man supports himself with his forearms on either side of the woman. This position requires a great deal of flexibility from the woman!

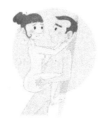

25. SUSPENDED CONGRESS

Lifting the woman off the ground, the man leans back against a wall. As he enters her, he holds her weight with his hips, shifting his hands from her bottom to her thighs. She can place her feet on the wall and arms behind the man's neck for more support!

26. THE SUSPENDED SCISSORS

The woman lies on the edge of the bed, feet just touching the mattress. She then places her left hand on the floor, supporting a raised body. The man then stands, straddling her left leg and raising her right, and penetrates her from behind.

This position requires a great level of strength and balance. To make it a little easier, have the woman's free hand hold or lock into the man's left arm or shoulder.

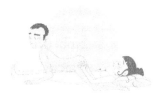

27. THE PROPELLER

While the woman lies flat on her back with her legs closed, the man rests on top of her, facing the opposite direction. Once inside of her, he moves his hips in a circular motion, as if to stir. This motion is often completely new for the man and woman, resulting in a unique stimulation.

It is best that the man positions his hands to support his weight should it be too much to place entirely on the woman!

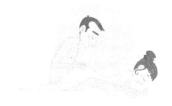

28. THE PRONE TIGER

Sitting with his legs stretched in front of him, the man sits with the woman facing away from him. She stretches her legs around him, raising her hips then lowering onto the penis, all while her arms are draped around one of his legs.

This position requires some flexibility on behalf of the man and is best transitioned into from a female mounted position.

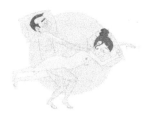

29. THE CRISS CROSS

Lying on her side away from the man, the woman slightly opens her legs. The man, also lying on his side, but perpendicular to the woman, slides in between the woman and enters her from below.

If possible, this is a great position for light touching

and trailing along the back of the woman. The distance should be too great for other additions.

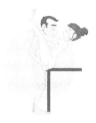

30. THE EROTIC V

While propped up on a table or higher surface, the woman has her legs raised into the air. The man moves in, allowing for her to rest the back of her knees on his shoulders. The man enters her as she wraps her arms around his neck, throwing her head back as he grips her bottom or hips to control the motion.

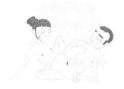

31. THE CATHERINE WHEEL

The man and woman lie together, facing one another. As he enters her, she wraps her legs around his waist. She can lie on his leg as they both lean back for support. After that, he takes his other leg and wraps it around her waist, locking it in place against his inner thigh or knee. This is a difficult position to master but can be extremely intimate.

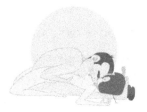

32. THE TRIUMPH ARCH

From a kneeled, straddle position, the man sits with his legs extended. The woman, with the penis inside, bends back and lays her head between his legs. As she leans back, the man follows, holding her close and bending with her body. The woman is then able to hump and grind on the man, having complete control.

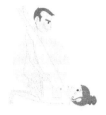

33. THE SHOULDER STAND

With the woman lying on her back, the two work together lifting the entire torso off the ground. The man should prop her legs on his shoulders as he raises up on both knees, penetrating her as she holds onto his legs for support and stability.

This position is best if you take your time and go slow! The penetration can be quite deeper than expected, so communicate!

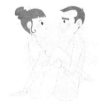

34. THE ROWING BOAT

Begin this position with the man lying back and the woman straddling him. Once he is penetrating her, the man slowly sits up so that they are facing each other, their legs interlocking. The interlocking of the legs is critical for this position, so don't be afraid to grip each other's legs with your arms!

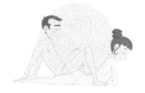

35. THE LANDSLIDE

This is another position specifically for a well-endowed man. The woman lies on her stomach, holding up her torso by resting on her elbows. Sitting between her legs facing the back of her head, he places his legs on either side of her waist. Tilting his body slightly for a good enough angle to enter her while supporting himself with his arms stretched behind.

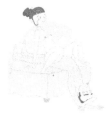

36. THE SUPERNOVA

The man lies upside down on the bed with his head on the ground and torso leaning off the edge, the woman straddles him and rides him. It is best that the woman leans back to counterbalance his weight. Also, a strategic pillow on the ground never hurt anyone!

37. THE SQUAT BALANCE

With the woman squatting on the bed, facing away from the man, she leans back on him. He supports her using his hands under her bottom as she gently lowers herself onto his penis. At that point, he can penetrate and thrust while grabbing her bottom.

This position is improved if the woman reaches behind the man's neck, putting some of the weight on his shoulders.

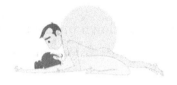

38. THE SEDUCTION

As the woman lies on her back, she bends her legs underneath her bottom and places her arms straight above her head. The man then gently lays on top of the woman with arms to each side of her body and enters her. A great addition to this position is a pillow behind the lower back of the woman, relieving density in the legs and allowing for higher hips!

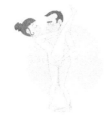

39. THE LUSTFUL LEG

The man and the woman stand facing each other. The woman begins by placing her leg on the bed, welcoming the man into her. Once he is inside, the two work together to lift the leg up to the man's shoulder while keeping the penis inserted. Stretching before this move is critical, allowing it to become an intimate and gentle dance of sorts.

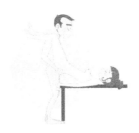

40. THE BUTTERFLY

Very similar to the Mermaid, this position involves an appropriately sized coffee table or lower surface.

With her bottom towards the edge, the woman is lifted up by the man from the hips, pulling her onto him as she rests her legs on her shoulder.

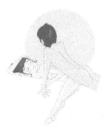

41. THE SIDEWAYS SAMBA

Making the shape of an "L", the woman lays on her side with her legs stretched out. In order to accomplish this position, she needs to tilt her pelvis inward. The man lays on her, putting an arm on either side of her, supporting his body weight as he penetrates her.

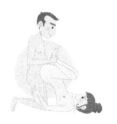

42. THE G-FORCE

The woman begins this position by lying on her back, pulling her knees to her chest. The man, kneeling in front of her on both knees, lifts her torso off the ground so that it is parallel with his pelvis. As he penetrates, he switches his hands so that they hold her ankles forward as she uses her hands to support vertical balance.

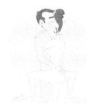

43. THE PROPOSAL

The man and woman kneel with one leg up, facing each other as if they are giving the other a ring. They unite in the middle, bringing the torsos together as the legs inch forward. The foot of the raised leg goes behind each partner. It is a relatively easy position that requires a bit of adjusting and practice to get right, especially if heights are not compatible.

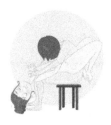

44. THE WATERFALL

With the man sitting on a chair, the woman comes and sits on his lap. While he is penetrating her, she leans back between his legs and puts her head on the ground or atop a strategically placed pillow. From there, the man takes complete control of the movement, touching and grabbing as he pleases. Be careful with this move! The inversion of the woman may be too much if done for too long.

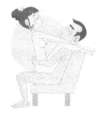

45. THE LAP-TOP

The man begins by sitting in a chair with something below his knees to keep them elevated. The woman sits on top of his lap, raises her legs, and wraps them around his neck. From there, the man lifts her up and enters her, dropping her back down with the penis inside as he supports her back with his hands. The woman is free to rock back and forth on the man.

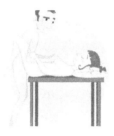

46. THE RIGHT ANGLE

Begin with the woman on her back toward the edge of a bed or table. This bed or table is perfectly level with the man's pelvis, creating a right angle between him and the woman as he enters her. Thrusting and movement on the man's part are not needed. What makes this is an advanced move is the woman's effect. After crossing her ankles behind the man, she massages his penis with her kegel and hip muscles as he caresses her breasts and clitoris.

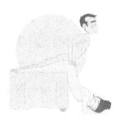

47. THE Y CURVE

This requires some serious abdominal strength from the man. The woman, lying face down on the bed, drapes half her body off the bed. The man lays between her, penetrating her from behind. To keep himself from lying on her, he pushes up on the bottom of the woman and holds himself level as he thrusts. Be sure to keep a pillow under the head of the woman!

48. THE STAIR MASTER

On all fours, the woman rests on a set of stairs. The partner, standing a few steps lower, enters her from behind. Be sure to use a banister to stabilize. An uncomfortable piece of this position is the arch of the stairs going into the shins or knees. This can be avoided with a pillow or by lifting the woman up by her legs. Be careful to attempt this position on the lower half of a staircase!

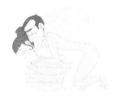

49. THE MAGIC MOUNTAIN

With the woman kneeling around a pile of pillows, her chest lying on the cushions. She should be able to put her full weight on these pillows without them falling over. The man kneels behind her with legs on either side of her, entering her slowly and penetrating deeply.

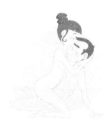

50. THE X RATED

Lying flat on his back with a pillow behind him, the man rests the woman on top of him. The woman should be facing the opposite direction with her legs on the sides of his waist, her arms around his legs. With the man's penis at a 45-degree angle to the surface, the woman slides, slowly, back and forth, each time almost letting the penis out before taking it back into her. Difficult to manage, but practice makes perfect! This is a difficult position that relaxes both parties while keeping them focused.

7

INTRODUCTION TO THE TANTRIC TEACHINGS

*T*antric traditions, similar to the teachings of the *Kama Sutra*, have been spoken of as if they only have to do with sex. Hopefully, by now, you can guess that there is much more to the teachings than sex positions and breathing techniques. However, Tantric practices have shifted since their original, more hedonistic approach to life, into something that is more connected and accepted by today's society.

Originally, the Tantric philosophy was an attempt to reconnect to rejected ancient Hindu practices that had become taboo. The hope was that accessing these different pieces of culture that had been banned would open a path to a deeper connection with eternal consciousness. The hope was to use the body as a connection to deeper consciousness and spirituality; the manipulation of which would elicit a more spiritual self. This included the heavy use of illicit substances: alcohol, marijuana and hallucinogens were all massive parts of the culture. Beyond the sexual aspects, there were also much more extreme practices like animal and human sacrifice, dark magic spells and the worship of violent deities. They professed grand benefits like immortality and regarded women as Gods incarnate, though their treatment of them was less than humane.

That was the old Tantric world. It was a lawless counter-culture focused on manipulation of the body through ritual and taboo. So, how much of the modern Tantric practices represent those hedonistic and magical ideas? Very little, thankfully. The modernized, Western adaptation of Tantric practices left most of the more colorful pieces back in the first millennia. But it did bring the good pieces—pieces that allow for the maximum intimate connection between two people.

In the West, it has become big business. The tag of "tantra" brings a sense of special, foreign sexual experience. It seems exotic almost. But in reality, it could not be more individual to the person. It is less of a foreign practice than it is the application of foreign ideas to a sexual experience. Modern Tantric sex and expression has its roots in yoga more than the philosophy of tantra. Everyone knows someone who does yoga. But before there is the act, there is the context. Introducing the idea of a Tantric relationship is a very natural and vulnerable proposal that can make all the difference in the connection between two people.

Modern relationships tend to have a barrier between the two people, often placed in the name of individuality. Practicing individuality within a relationship is often very important and should not be undone. Being in a relationship does not mean there is no more self. However, a relationship allows the potential to be more than one: more than the sum of two parts. Tantric practices work to unlock that potential and connect the consciousness of two people. It does not work to erode the barrier between the individual; rather, it looks to ritualistically circumvent it. Instead of destroying the wall and merging, Tantric practices are like two people digging a tunnel under it. Neither is positive where the other is, but they're looking. They unite in a moment, only to return back to their side of the wall.

Tantric practices are the shovels and seismometers you need to dig the tunnel. They take time and effort, emotional openness and clarity in a moment. The goal is never an orgasm, though that may be a piece of it. Rather, it is the connection of two souls into one.

Living a conscious life is difficult in itself, especially alone. To live consciously is to live in a moment unmeasured. Some associate it with the famous "Ego death" achieved through excessive hallucinogens—an experience of life outside space, time, and the self. Living consciously could be the subject of an entirely different book, pursued through art, meditation and knowledge. The Tantric partner works to encourage that pursuit of consciousness. Their job is to help you get to a place of conscious experience beyond the rigorous expectations of life. They aren't a safety net or retreat, rather they are a partner in exploration and a loving presence. Encouraging gratification, loving expression and giving are all their tools of consciousness and embrace.

What is shared when the tunnels connect? In short, love, energy, and connection to unlimited consciousness. Tantric union is an extremely vulnerable process and should only be done with someone you can feel open with. At the end of the experience is bliss and ecstasy.

Tantric relationships are like peeling layers of each other off until you get to the core of the other being, stitching wounds and memories of the past, learning and exploring with two people in a vulnerable and intimate setting. Your partner becomes a mirror to the self, triggering deep pain and joy simultaneously. It reveals intrinsic potential you have burning within you, independent of labels and definitions of the self. A Tantric relationship focuses on unlocking that flame and fanning it to be as strong and bright as possible. It is not something that can be achieved through a single ritual; this is not a single ritual. It is a continuous experience, day to day that goes beyond the bedroom and works to affirm the self.

Daily Tantric Practices

But like every intimate relationship, there is a sexual component. It just happens in the context of this larger, more connected and intimate experience. Tantric practices incorporate ritual into a relationship, allowing for a foundation that can be leaned on in difficult times. There are a few things you can do to incorporate Tantric practices into your relationship. See if they work for you!

1. FIVE THINGS YOU LIKED

This affirmation practice is one of the best ways to start the day. It takes three minutes at most, provides lasting connection and grounding in the relationship, and increases communication. Not only do all of these help with the sex in a relationship, they also improve the relationship overall by facilitating loving connection.

Very quickly, when you're in a relaxed moment in bed, at the table, or after a game, exchange five things you enjoyed about the time you both had together. These can be anything—simple and sweet, deep and profound. The important thing is that you feel connected in that moment, that each one is different, and that both parties participate. Doing this practice on a regular basis creates a foundation for mutual appreciation and affirmation, deepening love and connection to one another. It is so much reward for very little effort! Try it next time you see your significant other.

2. FIVE-MINUTE CHECK IN

This practice focuses on fanning the flames of the individual. It is a way to get your partner to tune into themselves, the moment, and the world around them. You're the facilitator for them and they, you. It includes the relationships, but primarily the focus is on the entirety of life and their being. As the one they trust and can be vulnerable with, it is a quick update.

In less than five minutes, provide answers to a few questions. These can be independently designed, of course. But a few good places to start would be:

1. How are you doing in life?
2. What's most important to you in this moment?
3. What are you spending energy on?
4. What do you want to create?
5. If any, what challenges stand in front of you?
6. Who are you right now?

Both parties share a quick note and update, no more than five minutes. They can be asked or simply answer a set group of questions. The importance is not in how the questions are carried out. The importance is that their answers are heard, both people are open and don't hold back, and both parties feel safe expressing their thoughts. Not everything needs to be shared! Respect and trust your partner, and this practice can only deepen a relationship.

3. SHADOW CHECK

This is a more difficult practice emotionally but just as important. The "shadow check" provides a safe space to develop and express problems in a relationship. It is designed to be a place of openness and vulnerability about the uncomfortable pieces between two people. However, it acts as a way to prevent problematic buildup and resentment in a relationship; it could not be more critical.

It happens on a semi-regular basis, or at least when you feel something 'shadowy' going on in the relationship. Designate a time to see each other in a neutral or public environment that might quell any explosions of anger. From there, you must respect the process.

Regulated by a timer, the first person gets 15 minutes to talk about what is bothering them. This is not 15 minutes to rant about how horrible the other person is being. Rather, use the XYZ formula. "When you do 'X', I experience 'Y', and it makes me feel 'Z'." It is imperative that both parties avoid blaming the other—blaming only begets defensiveness, which leads to more arguing rather than solutions. A key is to remember that you're on the same team. The other person is not trying to hurt you, the goal is to work through the problem.

The goal is not to resolve it necessarily in one sitting. The issue may persist into the day. But, working through it and developing a solution should become the priority of that next 15 to 24 hours.

4. CONSCIOUS SENSUALITY

This is much more in the vein of stereotypical tantra than the last few. The goal with this practice is to be completely awake and in tune with the sensations of touching, contact, erotic energy and lovemaking. It is another simple practice that brings more awareness into your physical space and intimate relationship.

Using a timer, do 10 five-minute interval practices of connecting with your partner, treating it much more like a meditation than a sexual exercise. Each of these can be broken down into different stages.

First Stage

For five minutes, sit in front of your partner and lock eyes, letting your body ebb and flow with the breath. Focus only on gazing and breathing for the full five minutes. At the end of the five minutes, acknowledge it ended before beginning the second five minutes.

The second five minutes is dedicated to a short, sensual massage of the partner's legs, arms, neck, and body. Both parties need to be fully present, not worried about time or discomfort. The focus should be on the giving and receiving of pleasure. At the end of these five minutes, bow, and switch places. Your partner should repeat the same steps to you for another 10 minutes.

Second Stage

After both parties have been massaged, the 5th round begins—kissing. For five minutes, practice kissing with full awareness. Nothing else, only kissing, as if you are both teenagers with no idea kissing can lead to more. Put everything else out of your mind and simply enjoy those five minutes of connection.

After the timer goes off though, the ball is in your court! Keep kissing or graduate to more sexual acts.

Regardless, this is a great practice for infusing connection more deeply into the sex! That's what Tantric practices are all about doing. This practice keeps you from quickly jumping to the next activity without taking in the moment. It creates structure to play off of and enjoy yourself through!

As you may have put together, these practices all hold a common theme of bringing awareness and connection into sex—converting sex into love-making and allowing for vulnerability that is required for a truly intimate relationship. There are many more practices to explore in these next few chapters. The next will take a look at personal Tantric expression and how that can be a core part of a successful Tantric relationship or experience.

8

SOLO AND PREPARATION
PRACTICES

*T*hough Tantric relationships are about connecting deeply with another individual, there are many pieces of Tantric teachings that explore something just as important: connection with the self. Beyond yoga, sex, and relationships, solo Tantric sex is the easiest to master. Beyond helping our sex life, it works as a medium for you to explore yourself as you might a partner.

The true nature of Tantric sex cannot be covered or understood through reading a text. Many texts use the metaphor of a serpent being coaxed out of a basket, rising up through the sex. Therefore, starting with the self to better understand what lies within you is the first step to engaging in Tantric sex.

Imagine the difference between a racecar driver and someone going on a Sunday drive. The goal of a solo Tantric experience is to keep all pieces of the brain occupied completely, granting greater awareness about your own sexuality rather than achieving orgasm. Let's explore, find a road you might never have gone down, and see where it leads.

Setting the Scene

The key to a good solo Tantric session is *time*. You need time and privacy—it is an extremely intimate experience that you don't want interrupted. More than that, you don't want to be worried about it being interrupted. Make sure you're in a relaxing, clean, comfortable environment. Lock the door. Light a candle if you like. Set the scene.

More than the physical environment, though, it is important to approach Tantric masturbation with an open mind. There is no room in this experience for low self-esteem or inner shame. You are alone and secure. Be inquisitive during your inquisition. This is an expression of self-love based on your own personal desires and needs—finding them is up to you and you alone!

Be sure to enter the session with a little bit of a

mental outline. Ask yourself, what do you hope to find? What questions are burning within you that desire answers? Are you looking for a new erogenous zone, or just hoping to relax? Making this experience intentional will help you understand your body better, faster, and have a better sensation overall. Leave the shame on the other side of the locked door and get to it! This is a light, fun practice. Laugh about it, if anything.

An important note—this is not the place for external stimulation. Porn is a great tool for masturbation, but the goal here is not a quick orgasm and be gone! This is better if it lasts longer, stimulates your mind, and builds sexual tension from the inside. How should you get started?

The first step is simple: Get comfortable. Once you've set the scene and done your due diligence, it isn't exactly off to the races. If you're tired or have tight muscles, maybe draw a bath or do some stretching beforehand. You want your body as relaxed as possible. After, make sure you're lying down, be it on a bed, the ground or a couch. Elevate your head, back and legs with pillows. Then, start with whatever makes you feel good during a normal masturbation session. If this includes lubrication, be sure to add that into the mix as well! But then, take it further with some Tantric techniques.

Breathing

The incorporation of a mindful meditation into a masturbation session allows complete connected-ness with yourself and the moment. Focus on your breath—feeling each inhale and exhale. Notice your lungs expanding and lifting your chest, the air brushing against the inside of your nostrils. Take your free hand and feel your heart. Notice its beat. Close your eyes and fade into the moment by focusing on the feelings, sensations of the body. You will fantasize and drift off. Notice this too, acknowl-edge the thought, then come back to the physical sensations of the body.

For experienced meditators, a Tantric meditation focuses the breath on an experience of each chakra. Sitting in a lotus position, breath in deeply through the mouth, letting the air dance down through the chakras. Do they have a taste or scent, or any discernible pattern? Have you been blocked, and if so where? Observe these sensations before clenching muscles near the pelvis, attempting to hold the last breath in. When thinking of the breath, caress your erogenous zones while keeping it at the base of your body for as long as possible. Once another breath is needed, take a quick sip through the mouth, slowly releasing the old breath through the teeth. Each breath should take 30 seconds to inhale and exhale, though you should feel comfortable experimenting with your own rules and limits! Speaking of erogenous zones...

Touch, Relax, and Lose Yourself

There are no rules here! You set the scene. If you opened up with questions, now is the time to answer them. Using a prop or toy is encouraged only if that is what you would like to do. Nobody gets aroused in the same manner; if you haven't already, this is your chance to figure out what does it for you. Be sure to touch yourself places that you don't usually go near! Find out what you and your partners have missed over the years.

Remember, though, the goal of this experience is not to orgasm. This can take the form of edging or resisting orgasm, but it is better if you simply go with the natural flow of the session. Regardless, though, all forms of experimentation go! Do you want to make noise? Go for it. Rock the bed. Pinch yourself. Figure it out! Find the hidden little pieces of a sexual experience that have been hiding. You are in control, within yourself.

Be sure to remain mindful and stay focused. If the thoughts wander, bring them back to the moment. There are plenty of things to pay attention to: How does it feel? Where? Keep your mind in the moment by grounding it to your feelings.

Finish

The end of a session may be an orgasm, but it also may not be. You're looking for answers, not a climax. That being said, an orgasm is more common than not. The finish, regardless, should be an awakening or furthering of the self. Not only will you have a better understanding of yourself after the session, Tantric masturbation commonly ignites a passion and sexual desire that may have lied dormant for a long time. Indian tradition called this the *kundalini*, coiled snake, orgasm—an awakening of a life force. It is the awakening of the serpent lying dormant at the base of the spine. It may not happen the first time, but that only means you get to try again!

Tantric masturbation and meditations are about harnessing sexual energy, opening yourself up to the possibilities, and answering the question, "What do I want to do? What do I want done to me?". The answers to these questions cannot only be explored through thought and mental games. They need to be put to the test. This practice finds those answers, unlocking a level of sexual clarity that you can then bring into any sexual interaction. Using these beginner methodologies will deliver a new person at the end of a session.

9

A GUIDE TO TANTRIC SEX IN THE ACT

*T*he importance of set and setting extends into all sexual experiences. Allowing sexual energy to flow requires coaxing. It needs to rise through the spine with comfort and intentionality guiding it. This is especially important in Tantric practices. The experience in total is a meditation and connection to the soul of another person and yourself. It is an intense, time consuming, and worthwhile experience involving the mind, body, and spirit all in one single act of exploration. Like any intense experience, it requires preparation of the mind and body.

The importance of relaxation cannot be overstated. But Tantric sex requires relaxation beyond a candle and a nice R&B song. Relaxation not only needs to embody the physical but also the mental and spiritual. This is achieved through a variety of practices: preparation of the body, mind, and environment.

The Environment

The environment should be a sanctuary. Whatever that word conjures in your mind is probably a good place to start. Candles, incent, or silk might be in the wheelhouse. Think about where you want to have the experience and make the area embody plush. Address all six senses—some flowers for sight or some strawberries for taste. There are entire Tantric playlists on Spotify, YouTube and other platforms that act to set a relaxing and enticing sonic environment. But this is optional. Any music or lack thereof that the two of you find stimulating is perfect. Wear silk clothing or something you find comfortable, or start naked. There are no rules! It is a sanctuary to the two of you, so do as you see fit!

Another critical part to Tantric preparations is what to avoid. In short, screens. Turn off the phone and TV, disconnect the landline if it's still in your life. Moreover, do not watch porn. Porn is not a path to connection. It stimulates and motivates a different experience between two people. External distractions of all kinds should be minimized. Everything you can do to keep the outside world out and focus each of you internally is welcome in the environment. Anything that might bring you out of the experience should be removed.

The Body

Preparation of the body begins before the day of the Tantric session. If you have not read chapter 8, skip back there and make sure you have gone through that experience. Tantric sex is not the best forum for questions to be asked and answered. Doing your due diligence beforehand is critical. Beyond making yourself aware of your own personal needs and desires, there are physical barriers that should be addressed to help relax the body. A bath or shower beforehand is a great practice—something that lets the muscles release any built-up tension. Sharing a massage with appropriate oils is a great way to achieve that connection and relaxation simultaneously, but light stretching or yoga beforehand is another great way to address these same tensions: making the body feel strong, yet relaxed, is ultimately the goal.

Both men and women can experience orgasm through breath alone—it is critically connected to all energies within the body. Tantric sessions begin with an inhale. As in yoga, Tantric sex is a form of physical meditation. It is built around and centered on the breath. After cleaning and stretching, the mind and body unify through a quick meditation or breathwork. Any practice of meditation or meditative yoga you feel comfortable with is perfectly acceptable. If unfamiliar, you can meditate in a few easy steps: Inhale, exhale, repeat. The goal of meditation is to ground yourself in the moment. Feel each breath roll through your body, watch your mind wander, then bring it back to the breath. Applying this mentality to the upcoming encounter does wonder for the experience. Practice it first. Your partner should be doing the same preparations. Doing them together can be a great way to get life's energy flowing through each of you, sexual or otherwise.

The Mind: Surrendering and Communication

Preparing the mind comes in two forms: communication and surrender. Communicating with your partner beforehand is critical to a Tantric ritual. Not only does it help overcome any nervousness either of you might have about the experience, early communication acts as the foundation of a bridge you're about to build. It needn't be serious, either. A few jokes here and there can be great for the mood. Make sure it is light, relaxed, and connected conversation about any expectations or fears either of you may possess.

Surrendering yourself is the first step in receiving pleasure, but it can be more difficult than anticipated. There are four main barriers to personal pleasure that need to be overcome:

1. SURRENDERING THE TO-DO'S

This is what you are doing right now, for the foreseeable future. There are no emails to get to. There is no chore or task that is more important. This is happening. The world outside your sanctuary can wait on you to finish up. You'll be right with them.

2. SURRENDERING CRITICISM

There is no place for shame in the sanctuary. These are real fears, problems and discomforts that can be addressed outside. But in this moment, in this place, you are here. There is nothing wrong with anything going on, nor is there a right or wrong way to do this. Clear your mind, be in the moment, and empty yourself of criticism.

3. SURRENDERING TO PLEASURE

Receiving pleasure is typically less focused on than giving. Tantric sex requires that you learn and feel your own pleasure as much as you revel in delighting your partner. This requires openness and connectedness within the self. To surrender means to witness and feel the energy move within you, allowing yourself to be worshiped and asking for that which you desire deepest. Allow yourself to not give. Be selfish and worshiped.

4. SURRENDERING TO THE PARTNER

All other forms of surrender boil down to this: vulnerability. To open yourself up to another in this way requires infinite trust and honesty. This is done through constant communication and affirmation. We're not just talking verbal honesty and vulnerability, though! This vulnerability takes the form of sounds, physical acts and movement. It is both subconscious and conscious, saying as much as believing. Decide to be open and vulnerable—surrendering to the accompanying risk.

Preparing the Act: Breathing and Kissing

Breath nurtures the fire within us all. Not only does it connect the different forces within us, it connects us to each other. There are a few different breathing practices that can be done to support a Tantric experience, but the first is the most important. Look into each other's eyes and begin breathing together. Breathe deeply, in through the nose and out through the mouth, and connect. Notice what happens to you, to your body, and your perspective of the other person. Take it all in. it connects the two of you while removing any blocks or interruptions that may exist. Beyond the synchronized breathing is a list of some more advanced techniques:

1. THE STIMULATING BREATH

Begin by closing your eyes. Inhale and exhale through the nose, keeping the mouth shut at a rate of three cycles per 15 seconds. Breath normally after the cycle ends, then attempt the same three cycles in another 20 second round.

2. THE 4-7-8 BREATH

While sitting across from your partner, synchronize this pattern:

- Exhale through the mouth, then close the mouth.
- Inhale through the nose and count to four.
- Hold your breath and count to seven.
- Exhale through your mouth completely to a count of eight.

Repeat four times for a total of four breaths!

3. THE COUNTING BREATH

This is more of a form or meditation in itself than the other forms of breath, so it is best if you have experience in that arena!

- Close your eyes and take multiple deep breaths.
- Let it flow naturally.
- Inhale, then count "one" to yourself as you exhale.
- Work your way up to five, each exhale being another number.
- Once you hit five, start at "one" again.
- Notice your mind wander, take note, then return to the breath.
- Do this for 10 minutes to become centered.

Breathing in its different forms helps to empower the body, connect to the moment and your partner, and lose sense of the ego. But there exists another way to become grounded together: kissing.

A Tantric kiss fuses these ideas into action—breath, touch, relaxation and coming together in one act. A Tantric kiss is for the kiss's sake, not a path to anything else. Hold together in that moment using a few easy techniques:

1. Gently touch your lover's lips.
2. Exhale while kissing.
3. Inhale while kissing.
4. Softly bite their lips.
5. Kiss at an angle.
6. Twine your tongues together.
7. Ying Yang—alternate between kissing tenderly then deeply and repeat.

These are easy and soft additions to a couple's preparation. Breathe through each kiss, fill and feel the other.

Touching

The building of tension within both you and your partner is critical throughout a Tantric experience.

Touching and caressing acts as its own form of communication between a couple. Tantric touching is designed to unlock the other person while building up excitement. Throughout a set of moves, Tantric touching follows a single rule: slow, light touch. You're an explorer, nimbly connecting the energy of your partner through the tips of your fingers. The mindset is not orgasm, it is worship. Touch facilitates that message. Hitting on the erogenous zones is important, but the rest of the body is just as important. Find a bump you didn't know about or play with a hidden piece of them. Take turns experiencing and exploring the other. For a more intrusive experience, there are a few key tools that will help connect two people.

1. THE YAB YUM

The Yab Yum is an extremely intimate position of meditation and connection. It begins with the first partner sitting, legs crossed and back straight. The second sits on the first's thighs and crosses their ankles behind the back. From there, stare into each other's eyes and breath in sync.

2. HAND ON HEART

Sit cross-legged opposite your partner. Take your right hand and place it on their heart as they recip-rocally place their right hand on yours. Close your eyes, feeling their heart's rhythm, focusing on the energy and the emotion surrounding the two of you. Don't think. Feel. Let the connection build between the two of you.

3. The Relaxed Arch

Have your partner sit upright on the bed or floor with legs straight out and supported. Sit your knees on your partner's lap, facing your torso toward them with your legs comfortably located. When situated, slowly arch your back, resting your head between your partner's legs, grabbing onto their ankles or feet. Breath and enjoy the stretch. The partner is free to follow the arch.

Guidelines for Tantric Sex

The preparations have been made; foundations laid. Both partners are relaxed and connected, ready to get into the act of ultimate connection. Before you go into anything, there are a few ideas to focus on in order to maximize the experience:

1. SOUNDS

The noises we make are integral pieces of the sexual experience. There are two pieces to every human: the god and the animal. The god needs to hear words of affirmation and encouragement, things that play to their humor, making them comfortable in the situation and keeping them open. Contrarily, the animal needs noise. The expression of grunts, exclamations, and moaning is often repressed through situational factors—a desire not to disturb roommates, kids, or neighbors. This is not the place for repression of any sort; be free, be loud, and make a noise you haven't before.

2. MOVEMENT

Keeping the movement slow and steady will win the race, except this isn't a race at all. A Tantric experience is not a marathon or sprint either. It is a nice jog through the park on a beautiful day. Keep the movement slow, natural. More importantly, pay attention to the feelings of movement between the two of you. In the same way you focused on the breath at the beginning, focus on the movement. This will put the brain at ease, grounding it in the moment and keep you from missing out on any connection.

3. IMPLOSION VS. EXPLOSION

Moving beyond the experience of the orgasm can be difficult, but Tantric practices are working toward another experience: an implosion of sensation and pleasure, sustained orgasmic energy rather than an explosion of that energy. Let it build within you until it is impossible to contain, then hold it back a little longer. Resist the orgasm and connect with your partner.

The implosion can only happen if the explosion is delayed. Both parties should try to not orgasm for as long as possible. The best way to do this: Do not think about it. Feel, sense the other person, and when you feel the orgasm coming, stop and do something less simulating that maintains connection. This process of on, then off, then on again is known as "edging". It is a very practical way to not only extend the sexual experience but a fantastic way to create a knee-buckling orgasm worth remembering. Even though it isn't the point, there's no harm in enjoying the side effects of the experience.

4. POSITIONING

In reality, any position can become a Tantric position. Tantric sex is not a question of where your leg is or how to angle to torso. It is not a technical experience, rather a natural flow of energy from one person to another. That being said, there are positions designed for connection and maximizing the sensations stemming from that connection. Those are discussed in the next chapter. Regardless, do not worry about specific positions. Do what comes naturally in the moment; being familiar with the moves acts as a way to know what is possible.

5. BREATHING

Losing yourself in the moment of passion and pleasure is easy.

6. TANTRA SAMADHI

Believe it or not, there is an experience beyond and greater than the orgasm known as the Samadhi. Once you've entered into orgasm and enjoying the ecstasy, bring it further. Lie down with each other, holding hands and fall into a deep relaxation together. The orgasm will wash over both of you like a blanket as you each fall into a timeless moment of connection. Achieving this grants access to a connectedness and consciousness beyond your own.

Notice that this chapter was not a list of "To Do's". There is no list to follow, only an experience to build for yourself. It is an extremely personal experience shared between two people. Nothing is wrong or out of bounds, so do as you wish. The important thing is that you enter the experience understanding it is not a quest for a better, more intense orgasm, though that is a side effect. Tantric sex is about connection with the core being of your partner in an effort to make them feel as you see them. The next chapter will go over positions that help maximize the connection between each of you through various Tantric positions.

10

TANTRIC SEX POSITIONS AND ENHANCEMENT TIPS

While the act of Tantric sex was desribed in-depth previously, the best positions to engage it in have yet to be mentioned. In no way are these positions rules to follow or checkmarks to hit. Seeing them as such would destroy their value. That being said, these are fantastic positions for finding the high-level, cosmic connection between two people that is possible when engaging in Tantric sex.

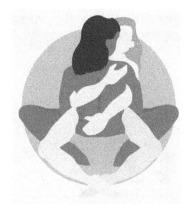

1. THE YAB YUM

This is the classic Tantric sex position, stemming from the breathing technique of the same name. Yab Yum is an extremely powerful and intimate connector between partners, taking the already intimate lotus position to the next level.

The man begins by sitting cross-legged on a stable yet comfortable surface. The woman then sits around him, laying her legs behind him as he penetrates her. After penetration though, incorporate some of the Tantric practices: synchronized breathing and locked eyes are the easiest to start. From that point, begin to rock back and forth, side to side together for deeper penetration. Create a union. For extra stimulation, the woman can tilt her pelvis forward to help hit the G-Spot.

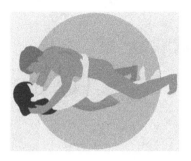

2. TILTED MISSIONARY

Missionary is the ultimate connection booster and a natural approach to any Tantric session. The woman lies with the man on top of her for some face-to-face lovemaking. Adding a Tantric flare to it means applying those same practices of breathing, staring, and feeling. If you're a beginner, do this for about two minutes before working your way up to longer times. After that, begin having sex while maintaining the connections as best as possible. To improve the position and G-spot stimulation, place a pillow under her hips!

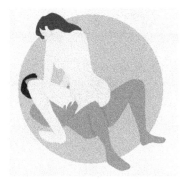

3. THE GREAT BEE

This position can be somewhat taxing for the woman, but worth it for both parties. The man begins lying back, the woman straddling him. While assuming the "cowgirl" position, the woman shifts her legs forward, resulting in a squatting stance over the man. The man lifts his legs to support her back and keep her aligned as she slides down on his penis. From that stance, she is able to brace herself on his chest while maintaining eye contact. The man can also hold her legs and hips to support her, keeping her balanced as he thrusts into her.

The thrusting in this position is deep but not fast, which means it feels great for longer—perfect for a Tantric experience focused on connection! It is also a good position to incorporate a vibrator into.

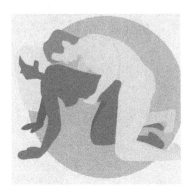

4. HOWLING HOUNDS

This position has a tendency to disconnect couples because of its similarity to the very animalistic doggy style. However, if approached in a new manner, this can be extremely connective.

Begin in the classic doggy style, the woman on all fours with the man penetrating from behind. Rather than grabbing her hips, though, the man should drape his body over the woman to create as much skin-on-skin contact as possible. At the same time, the woman should arch her back, throwing her heart forward and creating a pocket for the man to lay in. This is a powerful position that can create a sense of deep unity and trust between the two people.

5. PEARL HARVEST

This relaxed "oral love" position is the perfect extension of Tantric sex. It specifically hones into the ideas of worship and relaxation. All the while, it allows intimate connection.

This position begins with one person reclining back on a bed or chair, propped up comfortably. The partner then kneels in front of them, kissing gently before performing fellatio. The propped up nature of this position allows intense eye contact which, at first, will be awkward. But after a few minutes, it becomes second nature.

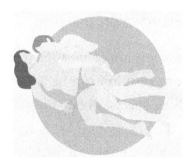

6. SUNDAY SMOOTHIE

This relaxed, calm and intimate position begins with the two in a classic spooning position. Because this position is so relaxed, it opens opportunities that others don't. Uniquely, this position is the best for simply talking. Having a conversation, opening up, and making yourself vulnerable are all key tenets of Tantric sex. This position enables that to happen.

A structured conversation around a game is the best approach, as the structure allows intimacy to flow rather than administrative thoughts. All of this foreplay is built directly into the intimacy of the position. When you're ready to start having sex, simply have the man slide into the woman, anally or vaginally. Then, it's a game of touching one another, feeling each other, and moving in unison. As the woman, looking back and locking eyes will only make the experience more unifying.

These are a few examples of Tantric sex positions. To reiterate, any position can be a Tantric position. There is nothing special about the positions themselves, rather the energy you bring to each of them. If you approach your session with a drive toward connection, worship, and vulnerability, and toss some Tantric breathing and eye-locking into the mix, you will have a magical experience. There is always room for practice and improvement, so you'll have to practice often. Oh, no!

FINAL WORDS

Sex is a unique experience for each person who has it. The decisions that go into when, where, how and any meaning attached to it are all very cultural. As such, sex is a core part of the human experience—a momentary battle between our biology and consciousness. It blurs the lines between society and the individual, man and woman, meaning and frivolity. Sex spans all of human time and has been a part of our collective culture longer than cooking or any other aspect of society.

Twenty first century sex has become something different from what it was in the past. It is not good or bad, though there are arguments for both sides. Rather, modern sex tends to only give those of us who live here and now a single flashlight to find our own way in the dark. There is an expectation of what sex should be, built by media, rather than by questions we ask ourselves. Finding the confidence and curiosity to ask them is the first step in a larger process. This book, hopefully, is the second. Educating yourself to a place of realization that there are multiple shades of sex—that before there were different cuisines, there were different forms of sex.

The *Kama Sutra* is one form of sex. It is not necessarily better or worse than the others, but the *Kama Sutra* acts as a direct parallel to typical western sex. Western sex is red hot, heavy all the time, happening anywhere and everywhere. It is the culmination of a love story in a single act or the beginning of a dramatic state of affairs. Something that happens in a fit of passion cannot be simplified or slowed; it requires an explosion to overcome suppression.

But the *Kama Sutra* takes a different approach. What if sex was a part of life, something that people did as they did other things rather than an obsession? Sex becomes less about weighty expectations of romance and more about the moment of pleasure and peace.

It becomes a puzzle to solve rather than a desire to quell. It also becomes a completely different color of sex.

Though it is only mentioned in twenty percent of the book, the sex described in the *Kama Sutra* is designed for pleasure. From the "Lotus Flower" to the "Slide", even the more modern positions are designed to help each person feel the moment, the other person, letting the pleasure wash over them. There is no room for shame or disappointment. Rather it is a methodology filled with questions of exploration and play, seduction and desire.

It talks about the importance of foreplay—how important the idea of 'play' is within that word. Having fun with foreplay can be the best part of sex for any couple. The building up of suspense and desire to the point of overwhelm is a fountain of youth that can always be tapped into. The *Kama Sutra* also dives into the art of oral sex for both men and women, not only suggesting it is alright but encouraging it.

Then there are the Tantrics, who realized an opportunity for intense spiritual connection. They saw a connection between sexual and yogic experiences, deciding to merge them into a spiritual experience of connection that could be shared between any two people. The Tantrics incorporated ideas of breathing and intimacy. Tantra is not a set of rules or regulations governing the way two people should have sex for maximum connection. Rather, as most things, it is a guideline to an experience—a set of tools in your toolbox.

The same is true of the *Kama Sutra* in general! There are few rules and regulations. At no point in the *Kama Sutra* does Vātsyāyana say, "Do these moves in this order and you will have an orgasm." Of course not! That isn't the goal of his book, nor is it the goal of this one.

Having read this book, you should have a set of tools to take into the bedroom. But beyond a list of new positions, there is a mindset with which to apply them properly. This mindset will not only help you properly apply these tools, but it will help you enjoy and release in the moments of complete ecstasy that come with sex and lovemaking.

Sex has the potential to be something more than the physical expression of our most basic animalistic instincts. It can be that too, and sometimes it needs to be. But that form of sex is only one form of sex. In the *Kama Sutra*, you find another. However, it does not end here. There are plenty of other cultures, each with their own sexual traditions, opinions, and taboos. Just as you might be willing or curious to try their food, it may be an eye-opening experience to try their sex as well. Best of luck!

CREDITS

Image Credit: Shutterstock.com

CPSIA information can be obtained
at www.ICGtesting.com
Printed in the USA
LVHW010536110121
676184LV00009B/433

9 781801 340182